CW01370729

My Journey

Sally to Shay

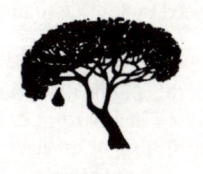

Shay Robertson

First published in Great Britain in 2018 by
Figtree Industries
3 Prospect Cottages
Snailbeach
Shrewsbury
SY5 0LR

Text copyright © Shay Robertson 2018
Reprinted 2020 minor amendments
The moral right of the author has been asserted
A CIP catalogue record of this book is available from the British Library

Some names and identifying details have been changed to protect the privacy of individuals. Events, locales and conversations reproduced from memory may be inaccurate. Although the author and publisher have made every effort to ensure that the information in this book was correct at printing time, the author and publisher do not assume and hereby disclaim any liability to any party for any loss, damage, or disruption caused by errors or omissions, whether such errors or omissions result from negligence, accident, or any other cause.

The book contains graphic medical images that some may find disturbing.

This book is not intended as a substitute for the medical advice of physicians. The reader should regularly consult a physician in matters relating to his/her health and particularly with respect to any symptoms that may require diagnosis or medical attention.

ISBN 978-0-9572390-7-4
Designed and typeset in Cambria by Figtree Industries
Cover and chapter heading design by Daniel Kevin Lloyd
www.danielkevinlloyd.com
Cover photograph by David Ward Creative
Produced by Figtree Industries

CONDITIONS OF SALE

All rights reserved. No part of this publication may be reproduced, stored in a retrieval system, or transmitted in any form or by any means, electronic, mechanical, photocopying, recording or otherwise, without prior permission of the publisher.

This book is sold subject to the condition that it shall not, by way of trade or otherwise, be lent, resold, hired out or otherwise circulated without the publisher's prior consent in any form of binding or cover other than that in which it is published and without a similar condition including this condition being imposed on the subsequent purchaser.

Thanks and Acknowledgements

I have written this book to help others. Whilst growing up, my feelings could not match how I was living and this led to confusion; I want you to believe in yourself and have the courage to be who you want to be. I simply want to pass on the thoughts and feelings I had during my transition to all of those who may be interested or curious about transitioning.

Thanks, first, to Julie, my partner, for standing by me throughout my journey and seeing me for the person I am: never judging, loving me, being by my side through everything - every appointment, every meeting, every consultation, my ups, my downs - and for making me the happiest person alive: without your encouragement, patience and love over the years I have no doubt that I wouldn't be where I am today; I would not have been able to achieve everything that I have without your help and support. This is something that I will always be grateful for. "You are the wind beneath my wings." I love you.

I also want to thank my children, Andrew and Aimee. I understand that this cannot have been an easy time for either of you, but you never disowned me, which of course happens to a lot of people, and about which I was terrified. I will always be your mum, I love you both very much, and I'm very proud of you. I have watched you grow into the lovely people you have become, and I am honoured to say you are mine.

To my step children, Carla and Aaron, I know it must have been hard seeing the changes, and I will be always be grateful for you standing by me and being there, not just for me but for your mum. I love you both.

To the person (you know who you are) who whispered into my ear, "You will always be the daughter I never had." I am still that person and always will be. I love you loads.

To my brother, Darren, we have had our ups and downs. I want to apologise from the bottom of my heart in front of the whole world. Thank you for for standing by me. I hope I can be a better brother than I was a sister to you. I love you.

To my dad: I was petrified about saying anything as I didn't want to hurt you and didn't think you would understand, but to my amazement you have stood by me throughout my journey and I need not have worried. I know this is difficult for you, but I know how hard you are trying, and to me that means the world. Thank you, Dad, love you lots.

To my mum: I wish you were here to talk to, I know you would be proud of me for what I have achieved, and I know you are looking down on me every minute of every day. I love you, Mum.

I am so happy and excited to be able to share my story with you, and hope it offers help, guidance, reassurance, and inspiration to all who start their journey, and also to partners and parents looking for information. Thanks to all the friends who have stood by me. I would also like to thank agent Judy Broadbent for believing in me and getting me out there to ensure that my story is told in my own way. Without you this would not have happened and I will be eternally grateful. Also thanks to Julia Dean-Richards, Figtree Industries, for editing and publishing this book.

I thank you all from the bottom of my heart.

Chapter One

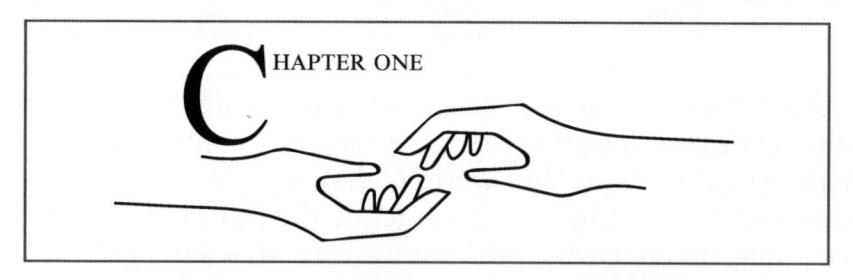

Sally Robertson Born 27.11.1970. Female

Looking back at photographs of myself from the age of seven or eight, it is obvious to me that I felt and looked 'different'. As I got older, those differences became more obvious and influenced how I felt about other people, and how they behaved towards me.

From as early as I can remember I always had different feelings. I never wanted to be dressed in girls' clothes or do "girly" things; most people would have believed me to be a 'tomboy'. When I went to the toilet I chose to sit backwards, as though I was a boy. I wanted to dress as a boy, and to have a short hair cut. I played with 'boy's toys', and I always wanted the toys that my brother was given, I had little interest in the dolls and prams that most girls were dreaming of. I was bought a pram around the age of nine or ten, but took it to a field and filled it with mud because I had become jealous of my brother's Scalextric. I liked cars, which I suppose stems back to having a racing driver for a dad. From a very early age both my brother and I were taking the cars off the trailer and sitting on his knee whilst he drove them.

My childhood was influenced by the jobs Mum and Dad did. We used to go away at weekends with Dad when he was racing. I was around a male industry and used to look forward to those times, really enjoying myself and feeling at home in that environment. My mum was a childminder and my dad was a salesman whose job took him to London every day during the week, so he had left before we were awake in the morning and returned after we had fallen asleep.

As I got older and started secondary school, I was a bit of a loner. Thinking about it, I only had two main friendships and those lasted until we left school, when we drifted apart as we followed different careers. During this time everyone around me started having relationships. They were childish ones, where they would just hold hands and peck each other on the lips, but I remember not understanding why I was more attracted to other girls than I was to boys. I felt that something had to be wrong with me. At the age of fifteen, I was asked out by a boy and only said yes as it would mean that I could spend more time with his sister, who was the one I was really attracted to. Throughout my school life, I used to get teased a lot, due the fact that I looked more like a boy than a girl, and because I didn't have a string of boyfriends. I was never part of the popular group and they used to call me names like 'lemon' or 'dyke', maybe because of my interest in cars and engines, or because people just assumed I was a lesbian. Whatever the reason behind it, this teasing made me question what I had been taught as a child regarding how people should behave in relationships and also what behaviours are socially acceptable.

When I was thirteen, one of the worst things imaginable happened to me. I was raped by my teacher, a person that society had told me I should trust. I confided in my best friend at the time, but decided not to tell anyone else as I felt they wouldn't believe me or would even think that I was trying to cause trouble in order to get attention. The teacher warned me that if I told anyone it would be me that got into trouble, and being so young and not knowing any different, I believed him. Sometime later he got another young girl pregnant and, as the story broke, he took his own life with just his car and a hosepipe for company.

I had grown up believing that you met a boy, got married and had a family, in that order. This was in the middle of the eighties and Margaret Thatcher was spelling out that a family should have a man and woman in the home. I felt lost and out of my depth,

I couldn't understand why I was different. Was there something wrong with me? Nothing felt like it fitted and, as my body was telling me that I was a female, I thought my feelings and attractions must make me a lesbian, right?

When I turned seventeen I started seeing a woman for the first time. This was a very difficult time for me; whilst I mistakenly thought that being with women and accepting that I was a lesbian would make me feel better within myself, I also battled with the idea of telling my parents. I thought that they would disown me as I would become an embarrassment to them. Looking back at this, it was ridiculous that I even thought this way, as my parents have stood by me through everything without question. I was thinking about leaving home as I wanted to live with the woman I was seeing, in a "proper" relationship. It didn't play out like that, though. By coincidence, a work colleague of mine that happened to be male approached me about moving in together. He knew I was not interested in men in a sexual way but, as long as we appeared to the outside world as a "normal" couple, he would not say anything about me continuing to have a relationship with my girlfriend. I thought this would please everybody and avoid upsetting my parents. Of course, if I had realised the damage that it would do to me in the long run, I may not have jumped into it so quickly.

So, at the tender age of seventeen, I moved in with my male colleague. The move led me into a battle with depression and I ended up feeling even more lost and confused. On the first night I thought I was expected to have sex with him, so I did. I can remember it did not feel right and it hurt. It made me feel uncomfortable and angry with myself for allowing it. After the first night we became two people who just happened to be living in the same house. He got on very well with my dad and was very pleasant to me; he did not moan that we were not intimate. I don't know if he was seeing someone else but we lived separate lives and I never really gave it much thought. Somewhere along the line, however, I began to feel inferior and angry. I couldn't understand what was happening in my head. I was not being intimate with either of the people in my life and it was making me think I was incapable of being loved.

I was scared of my own feelings and I think this led me to having sex with a man again. I wanted to try and become comfortable with the life I was living and certain that I was doing right by myself and everyone around me. These impulses led to me becoming pregnant at the age of twenty, which brought about a whirl of emotions. On the outside it allowed me to continue living my double life and it went quite a way to convincing people that I was normal and happy, living a "straight" life. Inside my head the demons I was battling were becoming more and more ferocious.

I don't know if it was the additional hormones because of the pregnancy, but I felt so empty and lost and thought that if my child was going to be a girl I would not want her; not because I wouldn't love her; but because somewhere inside of me I thought that a lesbian changing a baby girl's nappy would get me in trouble, or that people would think I was doing things I shouldn't to my own child. I understand now that people may think I was being a bit stupid, but these were the thoughts that were raging through my mind.

Because I felt so bad, when everyone around me was excited about the new baby, I began to be convinced that I needed to tell people what I thought to be the truth about myself. Perhaps if I finally told people I was a lesbian it would solve the crisis happening inside my head. So that's what I did. I told my work colleague, who took it really well as I think he knew that the walls were starting to come down around our pretence. He helped me move into a new house with the woman I had been seeing during the whole process. I also told my parents, who accepted my decision, with reservations.

Chapter Two

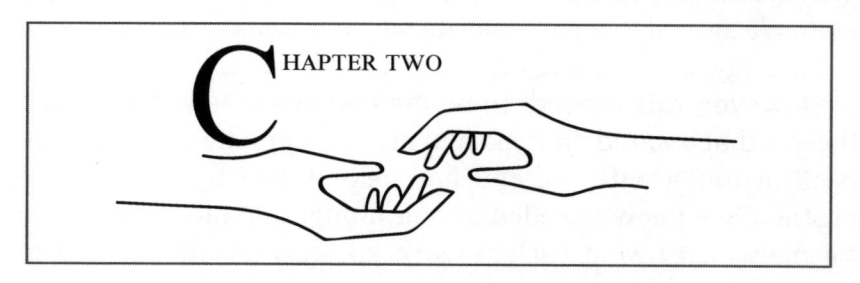

Sally Robertson – 1990 to 1995

The next period of my life – following the move into a house with my girlfriend – was fraught with difficulties and complications. My relationships took a turn for the worst and impacted on my family, friends, employment and health.

In 1990, it seemed as though things might work out – but not for long. My girlfriend and I moved in together, and were open about our relationship. During the first few years of living together everything went really well, my son was born and we were happy living in our little bubble. However, during this time, she had gone to a party and cheated on me with a random lad. I found out when I saw them kissing in the car. What confused me was that she stayed with me as if nothing had happened. Further confusion arose when my brother's girlfriend started making advances towards me. I knew it was wrong and I tried to fight it for a little while, telling her (and myself) it was not fair on my brother. But eventually I gave in; I just wanted to feel like somebody wanted me, it didn't matter who it was. Her relationship with my brother was doomed, not only because of me - she was also seeing someone else and ended up leaving to become engaged to him. She had played both me and my brother.

Feeling aggrieved that I had been let down and cheated, it felt like an opportunity when I had a phone call from my son's dad. He was just being a friend – ringing to ask if I was okay, so I told him what had happened. Lo and behold, he asked if I wanted to move back in with him and I actually said yes! It was to be a platonic relationship because by now I did not like having sex with men. We agreed to have separate bedrooms and I moved back in. At least my son now had both parents with him.

However, this was not to be the end of my relationship with the girl that wanted both me and my brother. She started getting back in touch with me and had also stayed friends with my brother. She knew I needed a childminder and offered to do this for me whilst I went back to work, so she was looking after my son full time and I paid her - a proper business relationship. As she needed to be there from early in the morning until late at night we decided it was easier for her to move in with us... As time moved on, feelings re-emerged and we started having a relationship again, only this time we were not very secretive about it and everyone knew!

We were together for about three years. I was suspicious so I followed her and caught her cheating again. Again I took her back, and for a few months we were okay, then, wham! it happened again. My brother told me she was seeing a lad. I didn't want to believe it, so when she said she was going out I followed her to a flat. I waited and waited till she left, then knocked on his door and spoke to him. I asked him how long he had been seeing her and he said three months. I laughed. I told him I was picking her up in an hour, and we planned our next steps. He got in the back of my car behind the seats and I covered him with a couple of jackets before setting off to pick her up. She got in the car and I thought if I parked up she could get out, so I chatted to her as I drove:

"Have you had a good night? What have you been up to? Have you missed me?"

All these things were coming out and he was in the back listening to it all. Eventually, after I had driven for around half an hour, he popped up his head and you could see the colour drain from her face. She couldn't get out of this one! She had been lying for the past half an hour. He wasn't very happy! I took him home, took her back to her mum's and went home. Panic struck me, as the following day I was due into work and now had no childminder, so I asked my mum, and from then on she looked after my son. He loved being around Mum.

Looking back it must have seemed crazy to the outside world, but we eventually got back together – I was obviously desperate for someone to want me. Me and my girlfriend in one room, my son in another and his dad in another room – imagine! He came down one morning and said he fancied pie & chips for dinner and he would bring some on his way home. That was in 1994 and to this day I haven't seen him. He called me about a year later telling me he had needed to leave - he and the girl I had been living with had been sleeping together. I couldn't take anymore. She was out when he called me, so I called her and asked what time she would be home. When she came in, an argument exploded! Once again, she apologised, and I stupidly agreed to a fresh start.

I went into the building society and told them I wanted to sell the house, but because my son's father was on the mortgage I couldn't sell without his signature and I hadn't a clue where he was. We carried on living in the house for about a year, then I went back to the society and did a voluntary repossession. I handed back the keys and they took control of the house.

My new start continued with a new van driving job, which I loved, as I met some great people. However, I began to receive unwanted attention from my boss, who started touching me as he was walking past. He found reasons to tell me to stay late and do jobs that could have waited till the morning. I had always tried my best at work, but it was becoming very difficult to stay out of my boss's way. During the day as a van driver I could be out of the depot a lot, but sometimes when I got back I found myself in very awkward situations. He would say and do things that made me feel uncomfortable - you look nice, smell nice, a touch, a look (usually at my bottom). I would make excuses to get away from him, like going to the toilet or to make a cup of tea, just praying another driver would get back soon. But dodging him was getting harder. I then got caught for speeding on the motorway and I had to go to court. I was lucky not to be banned but the points I was given meant I couldn't drive on that company's insurance anymore. I was told that, because of my dedication to the company and all my hard work, the company wanted me to become assistant manager. I was delighted, as somebody was recognising my hard work, and the company was growing and now had a few branches... Reality soon dawned on me and I became worried and sceptical. What if they put me in the office with the one person that made my skin crawl and deliberately went out of his way to make me feel uncomfortable? What was I going to do? Could I cope with yet another obstacle in my life?

I decided I was going to make this work for me and my son and that nobody was going to force me into something I didn't want to do. I would just try and stay out of his way. I discussed this with one of my friends, but at no point did I discuss it with the woman I was living with. It didn't take long for me to realise that things weren't going to be easy. About a week into the job, the boss came over to my desk and leaned across me to get something. He would ask how I was doing with my work, stand behind me, then lean on my shoulders and start to stroke my neck. I would just freeze and say I needed to go to the toilet, as I didn't know what to say, what to do or where to turn. None of this felt right. I couldn't say anything to him because I thought I would lose my job. I was breaking inside.

Things progressed. He would take my hand and put it places, and would lock the office doors so no one could come in. He must have seen this was upsetting me, but it didn't stop him. Soon came the time he led me to the toilet and had sex with me. I didn't want this, but never said no; I never spoke or made any noise, just went along with everything. When it was finished he left me there in the toilet and went back to work. I was embarrassed, bitter, crushed, tearful and very, very lost. I sat in the toilets and waited for my friend to come back, which was about half an hour. As I told her what had happened, she was fuming, but I asked her not to go to him as that would put me in an awkward position, and I didn't want to lose my job. As I am writing this now I want to punch his lights out. I don't think I would be as easily intimidated now, but this was twenty years ago and I have spent a long time blaming myself. I had been abused at the age of thirteen and abused by someone else in my twenties!

Within a week my boss (my abuser) fell ill with appendicitis and he was no longer at work; the relief was immense. I woke up happy because I could go to work and relax. I was truly thankful he was ill and no longer near me. I could be sure he wouldn't be walking through that door at any given minute. The company brought in another manager and later we became best friends - such a lovely guy and how a boss should be. We got on great and he led me in the right direction and taught me a lot. When he left I actually become manager of the branch and continued to work there for over ten years. And I would never have to cross paths with my old boss again - well so I thought.

Whilst all of this was happening at work, I bought a house with the woman that I was living with, all equal and in joint names. In 1995, I contracted pneumonia. It knocked me off of my feet and put me in hospital; even when I returned home I was still bedridden and dependent on her for a lot of things. Because I was now at home quite a bit, I noticed a pattern re-emerging with my partner. She had started to go out again quite frequently and even though I was struggling to do things for myself, she would be staying out late. Call it twice burned, but it crossed my mind that she was up to her old tricks again. One of my friends would come and visit me regularly. She would pop in for a chat or to give me a few magazines. My partner was going out about twenty minutes before my friend left and I eventually twigged that they had started a relationship! I was ill, hurt, sad, all my emotions were in turmoil. They even came home and slept together in the spare room whilst I was ill in my own bed. I was really struggling with my life and didn't know what to do. I still had my son to think of, he was always my priority and I needed to look after him. I felt guilty that I had left him out, in all my worrying about what she was getting up to, he was only five years old, and this horrible and ever changing environment was not good for him. The effect that it had on my mental health was not good for him either, something had to change.

Meanwhile, my girlfriend was on holiday from work for two weeks and I was still off work poorly. She had gone out one day when there was knock on my front door and it was my former (abusive) boss. I was shocked he was standing there: what was he doing on my doorstep? But, surprisingly, it was him who asked: "What are you doing here?". I remember it to this day but didn't think anything of it at the time. He said he was just calling around to see if I was okay. I told him I was getting better and then he left. I now know that he hadn't come to check on me; he had come to see my girlfriend, thinking I was at work. The two of them were having an affair. The truth had finally come out and she moved in with my 'friend' that she was now sleeping with. I wondered if my friend knew about all the other affairs she was having.

During my illness, I was offered a new job as a manager in a tyre garage. I jumped at the chance to take this new opportunity and a new direction in my life. I never returned to my old job, even though I had been there for many years. Something I found amusing was that my 'friend' took my old job. Was this so my old boss could keep seeing my ex, as he would know when her new partner would be at work? Goodbye, new start, and good riddance!

Chapter Three

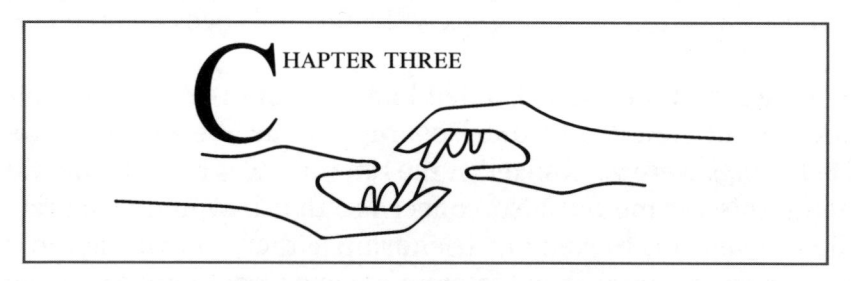

Sally Robertson 1996 – 1999

I had been through a lot and thought I had learned some lessons. It was 1996, and I was determined to start afresh and stand on my own two feet. At the beginning of this period, my priority was to buy somewhere in which my son and I could live happily and safely, then reinvent our relationship together. However, things move on quickly, and soon there were other considerations, too.

I needed somewhere new for us to live, so I purchased a derelict bungalow. It obviously needed a lot of work, but was finally something that belonged just to us. When I wasn't at work, I put all my time into the bungalow. When I was there with friends, we would make a fire in a metal drum, cook jacket potatoes, and just work. My son loved this time as he could see this old building become a home. He got involved too, hammering old bits of wood.

I met a woman (K) who was a delivery driver. She was a lot older than me and had two children. We eventually moved in together as this relationship was easy for me; it was reliable, comfortable and I was finally content... or so I thought.

In 1998, I decided that I wanted another child, a brother or sister for my son. K already had two children and didn't mind me having another one. I was unsure how I was going to do this. I had heard about IVF but I knew that this was very expensive and I didn't have a lot of money. A friend at work said he would help me out by being a sperm donor and that sounded good to me because I wasn't going to leave my current relationship. I set out to take my friend up on his offer, I bought test kits from the chemist to find out when my ovulation time was, as the last thing I wanted was to keep having sex with him until I became pregnant. I wanted it to be a one off.

When the time came, I called him up, went round to see him and we had a few drinks, dutch courage I think. We went upstairs. My feelings were very mixed at the time, as I was thankful he was doing this for me but also concerned that it wouldn't work. I didn't want this to ruin our friendship, either, so I was nervous on that count, too. When I found out a few weeks later that I was pregnant, I was delighted. This time around I actually wished for a daughter so that I had one of each sex, and all those insecurities I felt during my previous pregnancy did not resurface. I was older and didn't concern myself with what other people thought of me.

I had a very easy pregnancy, carrying on with my life exactly as before. At twenty weeks I went to have a scan, with my mum. The nurse asked me if I wanted to know what sex my baby was going to be: "Yes, please," I said.
"You are having a little girl." I looked at my mum as her eyes filled with tears. I was happy, and excited too. I would have a child of each sex, and my son was going to have a sister. There was an age gap of nine years, but it was going to be nice, I was looking forward to it. My parents never asked me who the father was, they were just happy for me.

When I got home, K asked if everything had gone okay. I told her I was to have a girl and she replied: "That's nice, one of each." And that's all that was said. Our relationship was more like a friendship, sex was very infrequent, but I was content. Sex was not a big part of my life at all; my life was my child, soon to become children, and to be honest, my work. I am a very hard worker, always going above and beyond in anything I do. I put my heart and soul into everything.

K never seemed settled, she always wanted to move house, complaining that there was nothing where we lived. My answer was to ask her what it was she wanted, because wherever you go you still have shops, grass, roads and schools. All I wanted was a settled environment. I hated the thought of moving, as obviously I had done it a few times. The bungalow was mine; I had fixed everything in that place, even down to light fittings. Maybe that was the problem, it wasn't hers. At least twice a week she would talk about getting somewhere together and moving away. I kept putting it off because I liked my place and didn't want to lose everything again.

Right up until a week before I had my daughter, I was working in a tyre bay. When lifting the tyres and the cars on jacks finally got a bit awkward and heavy with a big belly in my way, I took maternity leave. A few days later, I went into labour, and called my mum, even though K was at home. She told me to call the hospital and explain to them that my waters had broken, but I didn't have any pains. They told me to call again when the contractions were minutes apart. It was a couple of hours before any pains started and when I called them up, they advised me to go to the hospital. My partner took me in, and I was admitted to a ward because the contractions had slowed. I remember I was watching East Enders when K said, "I'm going to go home and get some dinner." I was a bit disappointed that she was thinking about food just as I was about to just give birth, but, "Whatever. See you later," I said, and off she went.

Around an hour later, the nurse on the ward asked me if I wanted a bath. They had put lavender oil in the water - supposed to bring on contractions. OMG, yes, it worked: I had only been in the bath about fifteen minutes when the pain was tremendous. I think my baby liked this bath and wanted to join me. I shouted the nurse and she helped get me out; they measured my cervix and I was very dilated. I was now in very strong labour, and my partner hadn't returned. I was on pethidine and gas & air, seeing cats jumping over my bed, and eating ice cubes like they were going out of fashion. I was away with the fairies. At some point K came into the room but I honestly couldn't tell you when, or when she left, all I wanted now was my baby to come. At 11.05pm on

February 7th 1999, my daughter was born. She was gorgeous, just like my son had been.

The following morning K collected us and we left hospital. It was good to be home. That first night, I slept on the settee so I didn't wake anyone up, and my daughter slept on my chest; it was a nice feeling. I had the bottle warmer next to me and in between feeds I could get some rest. In the morning, I got my son and daughter ready, and took my son off to school just a short car ride away. Then I came back home as my mum was coming to visit me. By now, K had another driving job, so, between 8am and 6pm, I settled down to look after the house and kids, and cook dinner.

After about a week, my partner again suggested moving. This time, I did consider it, and thought maybe somewhere else could be nice. I put my bungalow up for sale and it sold within a week, so we started looking at other houses. We were currently living in Leicester and now looked at places near Kettering. We found somewhere I liked, and within eight weeks, when my daughter was ten weeks old, we were moving in. The bungalow had been mine, but this time was slightly different. I agreed, as I was still on maternity, that the new house went into K's name. She had sold her house too, some of my money went into the deposit but the rest was used to furnish the house, fit new windows, install a blocked driveway and buy my partner a new car.

In our new home, we didn't sleep in the same bed. My daughter was always having tummy problems and cried a lot through the night, so the doctors suggested I had pen and paper next to my bed to note times she woke and what she did when she woke. This carried on for a long time, so she slept with me in my bed. We had a separate dining room off the kitchen, which we turned into K's bedroom, and she was happy with the arrangement.

For a while, I put all my time into looking after my children and cleaning the house. K looked for another job, and found one in a warehouse. My mum was the only person I actually saw anything of, as I didn't have friends apart from my two besties who were miles away. She started to drive over and see me once a week. We would go for a walk or into the town for a couple of hours and then she would set off home. I loved these times, as Mum wasn't keen on driving and seldom left the town where she lived.

CHAPTER FOUR

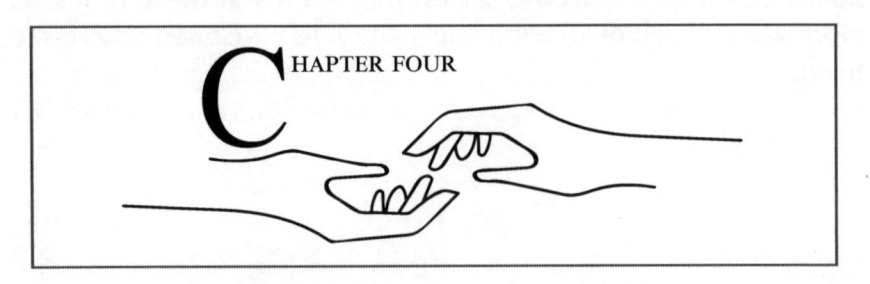

Sally Robertson 2000 – 2003

In 2000, Millennium year, when we had lived in our house in Kettering for about a year, K mentioned the moving thing again. I didn't get it, and was sick of moving, added to the fact my son had already attended three schools by the age of ten. When she came home one day and said she was selling the house, my face dropped. I told her I didn't want to move, but as the mortgage was in her name I couldn't do anything, it was going to be a bloody upheaval again.

My life sucked. It didn't seem to matter what I did, it was never right. I didn't have a house anymore, because technically it was K's; I wasn't employed anymore, because I decided to bring up my children and not go back to work yet. So, having once had a lovely bungalow, I now owned nothing. Having had a mortgage from the age of seventeen, working really hard to build myself up, I was back on the floor with nothing. Again, the fool word seems to fit. The only good thing in my life was my kids.

I contacted the social, as I was unemployed, and said my partner was selling the house where I was staying. Eventually, they found a house for me and my kids in the next town, and K stayed in hers. Mum came to look at the house: it had three bedrooms, but honestly, you have never seen anything like it. The grass was ten feet high, you could scrape nicotine off the woodwork, there was graffiti on the walls, the bath was smashed, and there were no carpets. Whoever had been there, had lived in a hole. Even the Council lady said that if I didn't want to take it she would understand, but assured me that if I did, they would give me vouchers to decorate, provide a skip and get a gardener in - completely my decision. I looked at Mum and thought, it will be hard work, but I'm not scared of hard work. She offered to come over and help me get it all done, so I agreed to take it on and began 'Mission Clean the House'. Two months later, we moved in.

K eventually sold her house, and asked if she could live with us whilst she found another house to buy. A year went by and when she found a house in Leicester, close to my parents' house, she asked us to move with her. I was tempted by the prospect of Mum being able to look after the kids when they weren't at school; this time, though, we agreed I would go in on the mortgage. The house was lovely and big, the area was nice, and both kids enrolled at the same school, which was literally across the street. I got a part-time job in the local garage and would take the kids to school, go to work, then pick them up and go home and cook dinner. For a while, everything seemed ideal.

K was never the nice step-parent - my son certainly didn't get along with her. She was always shouting or telling him off. Yes, he was mischievous and a handful but he was mine and we would fall out a lot about the way she treated him. I never visited my parents with her because it wasn't worth the hassle; she would moan about them, or they would moan about her, so I only tended to visit them when she was at work. As time went on she started picking on my daughter. She wouldn't let her get out of her high chair until she finished all her dinner, shouted at her if she was upset, the same things she did to my son but he was older and could answer back. I knew things weren't nice, but if I said anything, I was in the wrong for questioning her judgement. She was eighteen years older than me and I thought she knew how to bring children up, but what I was seeing was hurting me more and more. I started to object and retaliate, and arguments happened, I had been a quiet little mouse who never said boo to anyone, but I started to find a voice. I remember one night she walked in and asked, "What's for dinner?" She sat at the table and I brought her dinner over - jacket potato, chicken, cheese and beans. She looked at it and said, "What the hell is this? I have been working all day and this is my dinner?" The plate went flying across the table onto the floor. Both my kids were sitting at the table; they just looked at me. I walked over and cleaned up the floor, not saying a word. She got up and went upstairs, I got the kids' coats and we went to McDonalds. That night, she apologised, but things had become very stressful.

Something had to change because the atmosphere at home was not a happy one. K was part of a football team, and I encouraged her to go out and enjoy herself with friends from the team. Then, she joined a darts team, which meant I had time to myself at home. I guess I like my own company, pottering around, without any kind of argument. She made a few more friends, which made her a happier person and not so snappy when she was around us. As time went on, she started receiving a lot of texts, and I noticed the same person seemed to text all the time. I was curious; I told myself it wasn't that I minded her seeing someone, but I would be damned if I was going to stay home cooking, cleaning and taking all the verbal if she was dating someone else. Anyway, I think maybe I should have been a detective because one night I took the sim card out of her phone and swapped it with mine. I got all the texts – yes, she had met someone. I swapped the cards several times, just to be kept in the loop, but didn't say anything. Being a soft pussy cat had once again got me walked over.

I had seen an advert about training to join a lifeguard team and thought, yes, I could do this! The course ran for three hours every Wednesday night, and my partner said she would watch the kids for me as they were in bed. Whilst on the course, I made friends with a woman who was a First Aid instructor. She helped me with parts of the course I didn't understand, and lent me books. I started to speak to my new friend more often and she would come around for coffee and help me with my work, I started to feel a connection with her and to feel nice about myself again.

Each time I went home, K would be in bed, sleeping, or pretending to sleep, but I really didn't care two hoots by then. Having qualified as a lifeguard, I got myself an extra part time job at a leisure centre. It involved working late for a couple of hours; again K agreed to watch the kids in bed. One night, I came home to find the person she had been texting in my bed, and my daughter, who had woken during the night, sleeping on the floor next to her side of the bed. I hit the roof and carried my daughter back to her own bed. I was uncontrollably emotional, and needed to leave the house before I hurt someone. Cheating was one thing, but this was a new turn - my four year old daughter on the floor. I went to a friend's house and stayed on his settee. I didn't sleep but it got me out of the way. The following morning I returned home to find this new woman giving my kids breakfast. I couldn't be angry with her because this wasn't her fault and I was certainly not going to look like the bad one in front of my kids; she was actually very pleasant to me and I didn't know how to handle any of this. I simply got my children bathed and dressed and took them to school. When I went back to the house the two women had gone out, so I went to work.

I called Mum and explained the situation and she said of course I could go home if ever I needed to. I didn't do it straight away; I felt a failure, but couldn't bear to look like one. I wanted to look strong and capable, but inside I knew I wasn't. For about three weeks, I stayed with my kids until they went to bed, then went to a friend's house and slept in a bunk bed. At six in the morning I would go back to my house to give the kids breakfast and take them to school.

During this time I had been swapping texts and calls from my new friend, and she asked if I fancied going out with her one night. The thing is, she didn't just invite me, she invited my two children as well: I was really pleased with this. We had become close over the phone, but never physical. We went to take the kids out bowling but when we got there they were fully booked so we went for a meal. I mentioned things were bad at home and that I had made the decision to move back with my parents. The night ended and I drove the kids back home to bed. Once again, I went to bunk at my friend's house, hating being away from my children. As I lay in my bunk bed, I knew I couldn't carry on like this. The following day was a Saturday; I got my youngsters ready and set off to Mum's. I left the kids with her and drove back to my house to tell K I was moving out. She actually seemed quite shocked. I just took what I needed and after nine years, it was over, there weren't any massive goodbyes.

Chapter Five

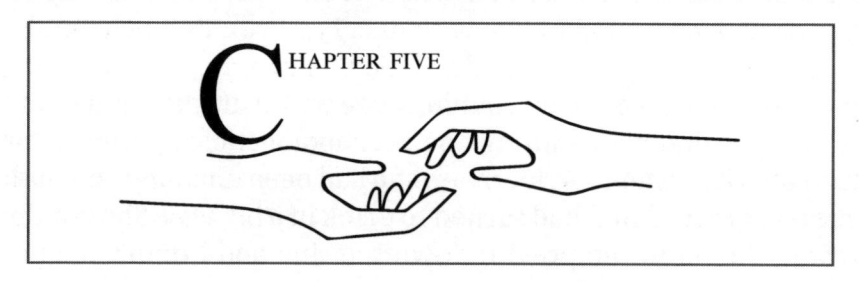

Sally Robertson 2003 - 2008

We moved in with Mum and Dad, which was great for Mum, as she adored having the kids. But I wasn't going to move them to a new school until I knew where I was going to be, longer term. I was texting and calling my new friend (M) and we were getting closer, but I lived in Leicester and she lived in Northampton, and her work on the ambulances kept her very busy.

Meanwhile, I worked hours to fit around the kids. During one of the daily phone calls we decided to take a massive gamble and move in together. We had only been out together once and that was with the kids, we didn't really know each other, just knew we liked each other's company. She started looking for a house to rent and finally found one in Northampton. I never even saw it until the day I moved in.

Because the house was empty we could move in quite quickly. I had only been at my parents' house for a total of two weeks and now I was moving in with someone else. I got a lifeguard job in Northampton, but had to give a month's notice where I was currently working, so for a whole month I travelled back and forth from Leicester to Northampton.

The night I moved in was nearly the last. I went off to work at 4pm on moving-in day, and M offered to put the kids to bed. When I got in at 11pm and she was drunk, I couldn't believe it. What the bloody hell had I done? I didn't even know this person - we had been on one outing and I had moved in with a total stranger.

She had drunk half a bottle of brandy. I didn't drink, I resented alcohol, my mum had been an alcoholic and there was no way on this earth I was going to live with one. I just couldn't believe she would do this on our first night. I didn't sleep, and the following morning I explained that I couldn't cope with a drinker, and didn't want it around my children. She was apologetic, apparently for the majority of her married years she had been unhappy and both she and her husband had turned to drink in a big way. She got the rest of the bottle, emptied it down the sink and I didn't see her have brandy again. Things got better and I grew to trust her. But something happened very early on I didn't like. My daughter was crying, and my partner got some saucepan lids and started clanging them together shouting: "If you can make noise I can make it a lot louder. Now shut up!" I hadn't seen it but she told me she had done it and my son mentioned it, too. That was quite a nasty streak, I thought.

 The relationship was generally a happy one. I did fall in love with M and she genuinely cared for me. We had lived in the rented accommodation for around twelve months when we decided we would get a mortgage together. I was now working in Northampton. I would go to work at 6am and work in the leisure centre till 8am, take the kids to school then go back to work for 9am, be there till 3pm, pick up the children again, then home. Some nights I would also work from 4pm till 6pm as a swimming teacher, and the kids would come with me and go swimming. We got the mortgage and moved into our new place, the kids enjoyed school and it was nice to have our own place again. Things were okay.

 People knew we were together, but there was never any affection shown outside of the house. We didn't hold hands or put our arms around each other, it wasn't that sort of relationship. To be honest, it didn't really happen inside the house, either, we just got on well. I could count on one hand how many arguments we had in nine years. We went shopping together, she worked, I worked around the kids, at home she would watch television whilst I did something around the house. After all my previous terrible, unsatisfactory relationships, this was one I was happy in, it was easy. I was content and so was she, so this, I thought, was it for the rest of my life.

But, in time, things began to change. She started to have small digs at the children. If my youngest didn't eat all her breakfast, she would be made to sit at the table until her bowl was empty. I didn't want the kids going to school on an empty stomach, but once my daughter was heaving and was still told to sit there, I couldn't agree. I would tell her she could leave the table and M would tell me not to contradict her in front of the children. My son hit his teenage years, and if he hadn't tucked in his white school shirt he would be told to dress himself properly over and over again; if he didn't get in the shower at the right time he would get shouted at. As time went on he would answer back. When I got home from work all I would hear is, "he has done this," and "she has done that". All I wanted was for us to be a happy family, but things were getting awkward.

I was not one to argue, and I let my M do all the disciplining, which is something I regret. I began to struggle to cope with her mood swings, and to resent her telling the kids off for the slightest reason. I remember her mum telling me that her own husband used to be exactly the same – how she left him and ran up the street carrying her youngest child in her arms, just to get away from him. M's eldest daughter moved in with us. She was a good kid and we got on well. We would go up the local supermarket just to get out the house for an hour. She told me she wouldn't let her boyfriend speak to her the way her mum spoke to me and the children. Her boyfriend agreed: "I think you need to get the kids and just leave."

When M opened her bottle or bottles of red wine on a nightly basis, the smell would turn my stomach: alcohol was something I couldn't relate to, and I don't like what it does to people. I didn't want to be around this, and despite my love for this woman we began to drift apart. One day, my daughter was crying and M told her if she didn't stop she would put her in a cold shower. When she didn't stop, she carried out her threat. I lost the plot and we had a massive row.

I was working away the following week and during one of our phone conversations I told her I wanted to split. When I got home, we talked, and although we didn't part immediately, it was clear we were on a rocky road to heartbreak and upset.

Chapter Six

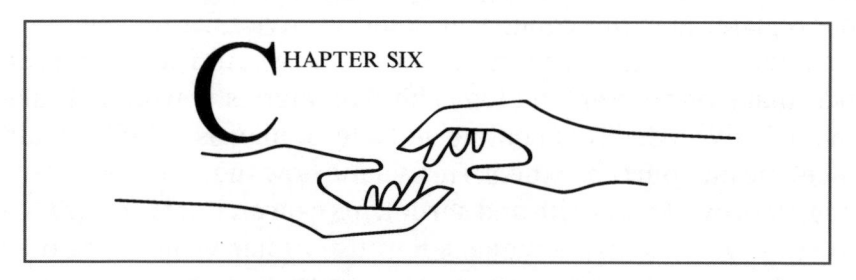

Sally Robertson 2008 - Mum

During this time, my mum, who I spoke with most days, complained of a sore throat. She didn't want to waste the doctor's time so just took over the counter remedies, until she started to struggle swallowing. When she eventually went to see the doctor, she was diagnosed with acid reflux and told not to eat fatty things. Over the next month, she lost weight, but I thought that could be because she was struggling to eat. She went back to the doctors and they sent her to Glenfield hospital for a scan. She was referred to Nottingham hospital for a CAT scan on the Wednesday, and on Friday October 26th 2008, the results were in.

Mum waited until I was home from work before she called to tell me she had oesophageal cancer. She had found out at 10am but didn't want to upset me at work. My emotions ran wild; the remote control flew against the wall; I felt angry, upset, useless, empty, terrified and tearful. Surely they had this wrong? Not my mum and my best friend?

I made an effort to see her every day, and bought some cream to rub between her shoulder blades when she was in pain. She sat on the settee and told me she was more afraid of leaving her family behind than she was afraid of dying. I told her not to be daft and that she wasn't going anywhere. My life went on hold as I searched the internet for a cure. Every spare minute would be spent looking at statistics, and finding foods and drinks that might help. I ordered some tablets from America: Mum said she would show them to her consultant and see what he thought. He said he had heard of them, and that they might help, but because they were not registered in this country he couldn't advise her to take them. He advised her to stick with UK procedures. All I wanted to do was make her better, and I was kind of angry she wouldn't take them. I advertised them online and a local man asked if he could meet me and purchase them. He told me how they had helped his dog, improved his health and shrunk his cancer. But Mum wanted to stick with the professionals. Because of her weight loss they wouldn't recommend any operation, so they offered chemo and radiotherapy.

I became very depressed, hateful, incapable, frustrated, preoccupied and cold. I didn't want anyone around me, even struggled to hold conversations with people at work. As for my home life, I shut M off big time; she tried hard to help, but I didn't want help, I wanted my mum.

It would be Mum and Dad's Ruby Anniversary on December 7th 2008. They had booked a holiday to Gran Canaria, but we were unsure whether Mum would be able to go or not, depending on treatment. For their present I bought a photography package for all the family. We had a great, fun day, with the photographer taking hundreds of shots. He said we could go and view them a week later.

On November 27th (my Birthday) my mum was admitted into Leicester Hospital for the first of many scheduled chemo sessions. It was also the day to view the photographs in Peterborough, so it was a busy day for all, as I was working in London and my brother was travelling from Lincolnshire.

We all arrived in Peterborough: I was there first, then my brother, then my parents turned up last of all – unusual, as Dad is always early. We saw them walk up to the shop, then something strange happened. My mum knocked on the window, waved, and walked off really fast. My mum never walked fast, certainly not away from where she was heading, and on her own. I left the shop and ran to catch her. She said she needed the toilet, and there was a supermarket virtually next door. As we walked into the shop she said something strange and out of the blue: "Make sure you put a sat nav in my coffin, so I can find my way." I laughed and told her not to say such things. She was very jittery, shaky, a bit like Billy the Whizz, not my usual mum. I had never seen her like this, it seemed as though she was on edge, but she *had* just had chemotherapy.

We went back to the studio, and were shown to the viewing room. It was all done really nicely, with music playing. There were so many great photographs to choose from - Mum wanted them all. We eventually narrowed it down and Mum wrote out a hefty cheque. Ouch! Her writing on the cheque was all shaky; she certainly was not right. We walked to the car and she got straight in, which, again, wasn't like her. She would normally give us a kiss and a hug. She even forgot to give me the birthday present that was on her car seat. I went over to her window, gave her a kiss and said is that my present? I laughed. She gave me the present, said: "Happy Birthday! Love you lots." I returned: "Love you, too." Then we all went home.

The following day was a Friday and I was back in London again. When I got home, Mum called me, and we chatted for a while. She also called my brother, and her sister. About an hour later my home phone rang again. M answered. I didn't know who was on the end of the phone but her face showed something was wrong, she put the phone down and said it was Dad. I just stared at her. "He has lost your mum," she said.

My whole body went into shock: cold, shaking, tears running down my face. I grabbed the phone and called my dad. He was crying down the phone: "She's gone, chick."

"When? Where is she? How?" I didn't know what I was doing or what was around me. I was pacing up and down the lounge. All I knew was I was going to Leicester right then. My son was out, but my daughter was at home. M took the car keys off me and we dropped my daughter off at M's mum's, and drove to Leicester. The journey seemed to last an eternity; it was the coldest and foggiest night ever, but I needed to get there fast. When we pulled up at the house, my aunty and uncle were outside. I kissed my aunty then walked in to see Dad. The police were there; it was classed as a sudden death and he had to answer questions. It had only ever been Mum and Dad, together forever; he would walk the earth for her, and she for him; this was just so unfair.

I went upstairs to see Mum lying peacefully on her bed. How could this happen to the most loving, caring, generous person in the whole world? I was torn apart. My brother came upstairs and we just held her, crying. I looked at her necklace and twizzled it to the front, to see the gold boxing gloves I bought her recently as a symbol, to get her to fight this horrible disease. I had just lost one of the biggest parts of my life - I have to be honest, I really couldn't cope.

After the weekend, I called my boss. He said I could have time off but I said I needed to work to take my mind off what had happened. I stayed with my dad for six weeks, driving up and down the motorway from Leicester to London each weekday. When I went home at weekends, my brother would see Dad. It was a struggle: my mum had done everything in the house since we were kids - the cooking, cleaning, washing, everything, whilst my dad went to work and provided for us all. He didn't really know where to start. These days, though, all is clean and tidy, nothing is out of place. Mum would be proud.

I became very withdrawn, burying myself in my work all day, then seeking refuge behind my computer when I got in. My son was eighteen and had left home to live with a girl with a child on the way. My daughter, now ten, was doing well at school, then coming home and spending time in her room. Downstairs, Deal or No Deal would be on and M would be watching tele from the minute she got in till she went to bed. When I vacuumed the settee, I joked that I didn't need to do her seat as she was always sitting in it, so there were no dog hairs. My relationship struggled. None of this was M's fault, she tried hard with me, I just shut off completely. I didn't feel capable of love, didn't want to love,

I wanted my mum. If I couldn't have her, I didn't want anything. I remember being on the motorway and getting close to the back of a lorry and just wanting to end my life to be with Mum. My boss would call me on my journey home just to make sure I was okay, and at times he would tell me to pull over. This was the hardest part of my life, my dad would say no one knew how he felt, but she had been the one who was always there for me, and now was there no longer.

Chapter Seven

Sally Robertson 2009 - 2011

A couple of years passed and M and I carried on, as most couples do, but things were no better. One morning, in 2009, I caught sight of a lovely looking woman on reception at the leisure centre where I worked. She was laughing and talking and had a bubbly personality. She looked at me and I looked back and it made me smile; I hadn't smiled in such a long time. My initial thought was that I was wrong to feel anything – I was a gay woman in a relationship; she was a very straight woman. Time went on and so did the looks. It felt nice, but I didn't act on it. When she asked for my phone number, I didn't give it; I was the swim manager and my number was in the manager book, so I figured if she really wanted to know, she could look it up - she didn't. After not seeing her for a few weeks, I asked her manager where she was, to be told she had left. I wasn't expecting that, but I figured it was for the best, as I was having feelings for a straight woman and could've ended up looking very stupid at work if I was reading this all wrong.

A couple more years passed. In 2011, I was sitting in a hotel in Croydon, scrolling through 'people you might know' on a social media site, when I came across a familiar name. I sent a message:

"Hello Julie, I am down your neck of the woods."

"You took your time," she replied. A smile appeared on my face and I hadn't even seen her; she managed to make me feel important, cheerful, free, relaxed yet strangely nervous; I got butterflies in my stomach as we chatted.

We started texting. I was still in a relationship and I was doing what people had done to me in previous relationships, I was being the cheat, and now I was going to hurt someone. It was not intentional, I certainly didn't go out to hurt M, but Julie was making me feel good about myself, something I hadn't had in such a long time. She wasn't in a relationship, but I knew somewhere along the line this was going to cause hurt. I tried to put my feelings to one side, for the sake of turning the house, the kids' schooling, my partner and my pets upside down; but I just wanted to be happy, and I was happy when I heard from Julie.

Meanwhile, my dad treated the family to a holiday in Turkey; it was the first time he had been anywhere since my mum died. I couldn't take Mum's place but tried my hardest to be there for him. I hoped my mum would approve of me making this my responsibility. My son's girlfriend was about to have a baby, so he stayed home. I really enjoyed it, but my partner and my daughter weren't keen. During the day, we stayed down by the pool, dipping in and out and playing on the slides, or went jet skiing and on scuba diving excursions: It was fun! M didn't like the sun or the water much, so she would stay down by the pool for about an hour, and then go back to the room to read, complaining of feeling unwell. My daughter spent time with a group she had met. Most evenings, I would go downstairs for drinks with my brother and sister-in-law, or walk to the nearby town.

During the holiday, I had been exchanging texts with Julie, and as it came to an end, I knew I had to tell M I had feelings for someone else. We landed at East Midlands airport and drove home to Northampton. I don't really speak when I'm driving and she was asleep, but I was thinking about Julie and how I could sort out my mess. We arrived home, took the suitcases into the lounge, and I put the kettle on. My daughter went upstairs and my partner sat on the settee and picked up the paper. I came out with it: "I have feelings for someone else." She closed the paper slowly, walked into the kitchen and returned with a bottle of wine. I explained I had met someone at work, that nothing had actually happened between us yet, but I did have feelings for her and we had been chatting for a month. I wanted to be up front. I can't for the life of me remember the rest of the evening, but I know she went to bed early and I texted Julie to tell her the news.

I now needed to sort things out. I worked away a lot, and my partner helped look after the kids. If she suddenly stopped having them I would have to give up the job that I enjoyed. I knew my daughter missed me and vice versa, but I had to keep the roof over our heads. We carried on like this until December, when it just was not working anymore.

I was seeing Julie when I could, and trying to juggle my work life and time with my daughter. On the odd occasion, Julie would come and stay in a hotel with me when I was away, and it was during the first time she stayed I knew my life was about to change. We were watching television and Shayne Ward was on. I was looking at him, as I had several times before, and I asked Julie if she thought he was good looking. I said I liked his hair, I liked his stubble, I liked the way he presented himself, and she just looked at me. The next bit was a bombshell.

"You want to be a man, don't you?" she asked. I didn't speak, just looked out of my hotel window, not knowing how to answer. The next minutes seemed to last for ever. I had mixed emotions: embarrassed, hesitant, unsure, but hopeful... the relationship had only just started and could possibly be over straight away, depending on my answer.

"Yes," I said.

"It doesn't matter to me whether you are man or woman. I want you for you."

I was so happy, so lucky! Where did I find her? I had been in two long term relationships and neither partner had picked up on anything. But, to be honest, I had never said anything, just had thoughts in my head that I didn't understand. I always knew I was attracted to women so surely that made me gay/lesbian, didn't it?

I spent that Christmas with Julie and my daughter and I was very happy. M moved out and got a place in the next village. I received a phone call from her mother asking what I was playing at; the daughter I had got on with told me she wanted nothing to do with me, and her boyfriend told me to pack my stuff and leave now I had made my decision. According to them, my decision was wrong, but they were not the ones living my life, I needed to do this for me.

I kept the house for a while, living there with my daughter and the dogs. Julie introduced me to her children and their father - they were still good friends after five years apart. We all got on really well. The three elder children were similar in age and had left home, whereas my youngest was twelve. After a while, Julie's ex was looking for somewhere to live, so he moved into my spare room and we got on like best buds. Eventually, I moved in with Julie and took my daughter with me. I loved my new relationship. Julie was very different, very loving, wanting the holding hands, the cuddles, the closeness. I had not done this before, it was all quite strange, but in a nice way. The affection was certainly there, it's like she wanted me close.

We hadn't spoken much about that initial question she asked about me wanting to be a man. It was really strange, and I still couldn't understand how someone who had known me for such a short time could see so deep, to the way I had felt for as long as I could remember. There were so many pointers, looking back over the years: the dressing like a boy, wanting a boy's anatomy, having my hair cut short, feeling different, not fitting in, only wanting boys' toys, being unhappy, hating my body, strapping down my chest so it couldn't be seen, and attraction to women. I even had a poster of Tom Cruise on my bedroom wall, not because I was attracted to him, but because I had wanted to look like him. I sat on the toilet backwards to pee like a man, and when having sex I would think I was a man. I never discussed this with partners, just liked thinking it.

Julie and I had a great life, always doing things together, going places together, sharing everything she was interested in, everything I do and vice versa. She is very much a family person and loves her family around her. I was still working away a lot at that time, but we got my daughter a key so she could get in after school. My daughter liked Julie, too. Whereas before, I would come in and start doing cleaning or washing, as if there was always something that needed doing before I could relax, as time moved on, things changed. Now, I was sitting down, watching television with Julie and my daughter most evenings, enjoying time with my family.

One evening, we were watching a reality tv programme I had never seen before, and there was someone called Luke A (Anderson) on the show. I started to watch him, his mannerisms, the way he spoke. He was having a conversation with a group of people, and during this conversation he revealed that he used to be a woman. He was Transgender. I got out my phone and googled the word "Transgender".

Trans

Transgender, or Trans, describes a person whose gender identity differs from the one they were born with. There is no single explanation for why some people are transgender. Transgender people may identify as male or female, or something else. Transgender people may express gender identity or change gender by changing names, behaviour, pronouns or appearance. Some transgender people undergo medical transition, using prescribed hormones and/or surgery. Someone who was labelled a 'boy' at birth who feels they are really a girl would be called a trans woman. If someone was labelled a 'girl' at birth, and they feel they are male, they would be called a trans man. Someone whose appearance or behaviour is gender-nonconforming may not identify as a transgender person. Gender Dysphoria is a condition in which there is a mismatch between the preferred gender role and that denoted by sexual characteristics. The gender dysphoric person is not necessarily transsexual. She-males, transgenderists, gender transients and transvestites may exhibit gender dysphoria. Gender dysphoria may cause people to act in a way contrary to their upbringing and socialisation, a way at variance with their apparent sex, which may lead to them being ostracised and disadvantaged.

Transgender people may become aware of their transgender identity at any age, with some tracing identities and feelings back to earliest memories of not fitting in. Others become aware of transgender feelings, while others struggle with shame or confusion. Those who transition later in life may have struggled to fit in, but later face dissatisfaction. Some transgender people, transsexuals in particular, experience intense dissatisfaction with their sex assigned at birth, physical sex characteristics, or the gender role associated with that sex and often seek gender-affirming treatments.

Transitioning is complex and may involve transition to a gender neither traditionally male nor female. People who transition often start by expressing their preferred gender in 'safe' situations, then work up to living full time as their preferred gender by making changes a little at a time. Common social changes made by transgender people include adopting the appearance of the desired sex through changes in clothing and grooming, adopting a new name, changing sex designation on identity documents, using hormone therapy treatment, and/or undergoing medical procedures that modify their body to conform with their gender identity. Many factors determine how individuals wish to live and express gender identity. Early stages of transition can be difficult for the individual, and hard for other people to accept. The person will be vulnerable and may feel awkward. Hormonal treatment is initially given. Practice, hormones and increased confidence will help the person settle into a new life.

A qualified mental health professional can provide guidance and care for transgender people and referrals to other helping professionals. Peer support groups and transgender community organisations also help. The World Professional Association for Transgender Health (WPATH), a professional organisation devoted to the treatment of transgender people, publishes The Standards of Care for Gender Identity Disorders. Popular culture, academia and science adapt as awareness, knowledge and openness about transgender people and experiences grow. Patients who wish to have gender reassignment should first have a complete and thorough psychiatric evaluation. They must have a stable personality, have lived in the chosen gender for a least one year and ideally have been fully employed during this period. It is the duty of the psychiatrist to determine whether the patient will be accepted in society in the new gender role. It is also important that the patient has reasonable expectations of the outcome of reassignment surgery to avoid disappointment.

Chapter Eight

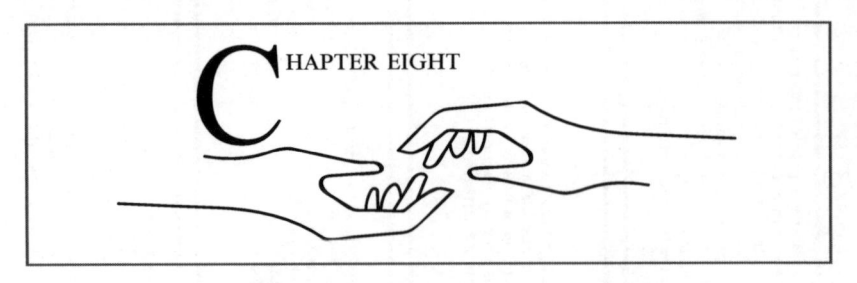

From Sally to Shay – First Moves

I wouldn't say it had anything to do with genetic influences or early experiences, and I didn't suddenly realise I wanted to be a boy. The feelings have always been there, I just didn't know what the feelings were. I had only heard of gay and straight, and as I was a woman who fancied women, not men, I thought that meant I was gay. Basically, I am my own person and do and feel as I choose. According to society, now I would be straight, but do these labels mean anything? I read everything I could, but found it very hard - I could find loads of stuff for men becoming women but not a great deal for women becoming men. There was online information, and images and stuff on social media, but some were out-dated, and I didn't know what to believe. I chatted with Julie and showed her what I found, and she said: "Let's book an appointment with the doctor."

I called the surgery and they made me an appointment. The week-long wait seemed forever. We went to the appointment, I told the GP I wasn't happy with myself and described how I was feeling. He didn't know a great deal about it and told me he would have to contact someone else and get back to me.

Eight months later I had heard nothing, so I made another appointment. This time I printed off gender dysphoria paperwork for the GP to read - kind of instructions for a GP presented with a candidate like myself. When we saw him, the doctor admitted he had forgotten to follow up my case. My heart sank; all my life I had waited to find the real me, and because he didn't understand, my doctor had forgotten about me. He apologised and looked through the paperwork I had handed him, it even gave a list of gender clinics that GPs could refer to. Now I felt the ball was rolling, and I left the surgery with a smile as he assured me he would move things for me. I just had to wait for a letter from a gender consultant.

After about four months I received a letter from a gender mental health clinic in Daventry, arranging an assessment. I was ecstatic, delighted, couldn't believe it, I was on the journey I had waited so long for. We turned up at my appointment to be met by a very lovely chap who made me and my partner feel at ease. After years of keeping this wrapped up inside me, it was good to talk about how I felt my world was opening up. The appointment lasted an hour and a half; I had so many questions I needed answering and the doctor needed to make sure this was not just a whim. I needed him to understand this was what I really wanted, but he was assessing whether I had gender dysphoria. He asked a lot of questions about my life, my childhood, my parents and family, about virtually everything. He asked about the journeys I had already been on, my feelings and my thoughts, and he made notes the whole time. I was very nervous; if he thought I didn't meet his criteria I couldn't go any further, so, I remember thinking, my life was now in his hands. He told me I had to change my name on all documents and bring proof of my name change in with me at my next appointment. He asked if there was a name I would like. To be honest I hadn't thought about it. I asked him what his first name was, and he said Bryan, I wasn't too keen on that, but I did say Ryan was quite nice, then the conversation moved on. It was getting close to the end of the appointment when the doctor finally said: "Yes, I agree, you have gender dysphoria, I will put you forward for a second opinion." I could have cried with happiness; this is just what I wanted. But my heart also sank slightly as I didn't know I needed a second opinion. What if the next person didn't agree?

Time rolled around and three months later the next appointment letter dropped on my mat – addressed to Ryan Robertson! I was not amused, I hadn't agreed to this name. Both my children saw the letter and asked who Ryan was, which was when I had to explain things to them. They were okay; I wasn't expecting to have to explain because of a letter, but at least it was out now.

Excitement and panic set in. We went to see the second consultant and just like the first, he was chatty and pleasant. He asked a lot of the same questions and we chatted for around an hour before he said that he agreed with the prognosis. That was it! I was finally starting my journey for real, with the backing of two consultants and, of course, my beautiful partner. This wasn't just my journey, it was hers too, she would be with me through everything and things were going to change. I did worry at the beginning that she might not cope with me changing, and I hoped our relationship wouldn't suffer, but that shouldn't have crossed my mind really as she was the one who had seen the real me. The consultant told me he would prescribe testosterone gel, but I had to have a medical first, with a different person at the clinic. Again, I felt disappointed, as it was dragging out and I just wanted to get started.

A week later, the doctor I saw on my first referral was to carry out my medical. It felt like a lifetime since I had seen him the first time. I was waiting for the go-ahead to start with the testosterone gel and hopefully be referred for my top surgery (double mastectomy). The waiting room was empty, we both sat patiently. My appointment was scheduled for 3pm; it was now 3.15pm and no one had called me in. I was eventually called at 3.30pm. The consultant read through my notes, then said that, as he was running late, he couldn't do my medical that day. He would get me back in again for a fifteen minute appointment. I was devastated to say the least. I had waited for this for so long, and it just was not happening! I left his office feeling very down, now I must wait yet again.

On 15th July 2014, we arrived at the second appointment for my medical. After waiting for over half an hour, I was really on edge in case it didn't go ahead. Eventually, I was called in. We sat down and the doctor re-read my notes. He asked how I was, did some measurements, weighed me, took my blood pressure, had a look at my arms, legs, stomach and back and said I needed to lose some weight as they would only consider me for surgery if I had a BMI of below 30 - mine was currently 34. He then asked me to go to the couch, remove my clothing, but leave on my underwear. YES, it's happening, I thought, and smiled to myself. After about ten minutes he declared that everything was okay. He checked my E.C.G. and said that was good, too. I was given the all clear to start the testosterone. I was ecstatic! Words cannot express how happy I was feeling. I thought I was going to be given the testosterone there and then, but was told my own GP would prescribe the gel, and also the prostap injection to switch off female hormones. Okay, I thought, I have waited this long, getting an appointment at the surgery will be plain-sailing. I asked if I could be referred for top surgery. The consultant had previously said I could be looking at surgery early in the summer, now he talked about October/November. Again, disappointment washed over me. The doctor said he would write to my GP with my care plan and that I would receive a copy too.

The beginning of August arrived, and I had not heard anything. I rang my GP's surgery just in case my letter had gone astray, but they hadn't received anything either. I gave it a few more days. On the 10th August 2014, the surgery still hadn't received anything, so, upset and fuming at the same time, I called the gender clinic. They said someone would return my call. That afternoon, my telephone rang and a very apologetic lady from the clinic told me my consultant had been on annual leave for two weeks, and then his secretary went on annual leave for two weeks, so although my care plan had been completed it had been put aside and not sent out to me or my GP. The apologetic lady from the clinic promised she would post the plan that night, and would fax a copy to my GP's surgery so they could have it straight away. I left it an hour then called my surgery. The surgery manager confirmed he had received the fax and would contact the pharmacy next door to make sure they ordered in my medication and to find out when it would be in. He called me back within the hour to say it would take a week to get my medication, so he had booked me an appointment for 20th August 2014. I was grateful to everyone, but felt like everything was in slow motion and my life continued to be on hold.

Chapter Nine

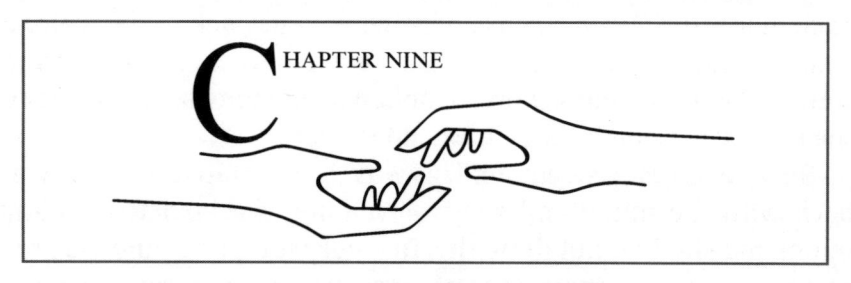

From Sally to Shay – Big T

Thursday morning, 20th August 2014 - my big T day had arrived! I was excited but nervous, too. I hate injections but it's what I wanted. Julie and I set off for the doctors, Julie asked me twice that morning, was I one hundred percent sure? Yes, sure, I had not waited this long and seen consultant after consultant just for the fun of it. This seemed like one long journey already, and it was only the beginning. I knew she had my best interests at heart and she tells me all the time she loves me unconditionally, man or woman; she loves me for the person I am; she will stand by me whatever decision I make. As we walked towards the surgery she looked at me and said, "Goodbye Sally." I looked at her and smiled. Then, we were at the surgery, sitting in the waiting room, my hands sweating, feeling nervous at the thought of a needle. I told myself I needed to get over this, as I would be having injections and regular blood tests for the rest of my life.

We were called in by the nurse at 8.30am. She asked if I had my medication with me: instant heart drop, why would I have it? The surgery organised it, made the appointment and rang to tell me the medication was in; if I knew I had to collect it I would have been there the day it came in. The nurse searched my records, they had ordered it, it was in stock, they had just not collected it from the pharmacy. Why couldn't things go right for me? The nurse told me not to worry, I think she could see the disappointed look on my face, and she left the room. When she came back in, she asked me if I could wait around for the pharmacy to open at 9am. If I nipped and collected the medication, she would fit me back in. Result! With a sense of relief, I went back to the waiting room. That thirty minutes dragged. I walked to the pharmacy and returned with my medication. I looked inside the bag: oh my days, the packet the needle was in was massive!

Now I was *really* sweating. This was the prostap injection. I was back with the nurse and she was reading the instructions and telling me she had not done this in a very long time and was not quite sure where to inject me. If I was nervous beforehand, I was now petrified. The nurse seemed to take forever to walk towards me; she was being friendly, talking to me, and making me smile... before I knew it she had done it, the only thing I could feel was the cotton wool being pressed over the injected site. I can cope with this, I thought. I had such a feeling of achievement. We walked out of the surgery, injection done and testosterone gel in hand. Julie turned to me, full of emotion, hugged me, gave me a kiss and said: "Hello, Shay".

From that point on, my periods stopped. For the next three months, I had a monthly injection, then went onto something called prostap 3, a three monthly injection to reduce my oestrogen and build up my testosterone, before I had a hysterectomy. As well as this, I was given the testogel (testosterone), which is a small sachet you rub on daily. There are different variations of testosterone but this was the one the clinic said was best for me.

The doctor had explained that the gel had to be rubbed into my shoulders and the tops of my arms or thighs after a shower every morning and it would be absorbed into my body throughout the day. He advised me to put a t shirt on straight after applying the gel as we didn't want Julie getting it on her! As, I guess, it is like going through adolescence again, the changes in hormone levels can mean you get very spotty - well I did, and I can only speak from experience. The gel is a very sticky substance but absorbs quickly. Regular blood tests monitor changes in hormone levels, so things can be adjusted if necessary.

Not all trans men choose to start Hormone Replacement Therapy (or HRT) for many reasons including cost or that their body can't accept "T"(androgen sensitivity), which does not make them any less men or transgender. Transgender males have a lot of luck when it comes to testosterone, also called "T", as it is very powerful really changes the body over time, unlike much milder oestrogen used for MTF's. Testosterone makes your body look and feel more masculine by: adjusting the fat distribution causing the fat to move off your hips, buttocks, thighs, and (slightly) chest, and moving it onto your stomach (you will not lose fat, just redistribute, so it is important to continue to exercise to lose weight). Increasing muscle definition (if you work out, it is not going to make you buff if you are a couch potato), broadening the shoulders, and perhaps thickening the hands and feet (may make them wider because of cartilage growth but no guarantee). The increased muscle definition and fat movement usually squares out the face (if you are under 21, you may grow an Adam's apple as well). Guys can lose fat quicker because they can gain muscle more easily(which burns a lot of fat) and thus you should be able to lose some of that stomach fat eventually (however you will gain a lot of weight first from becoming much hungrier and again you can't lose weight on Testosterone just sitting around, you must get your metabolism going regardless of your gender). Most men report feeling a lot stronger soon after going on testosterone. Increased body hair growth as well as facial hair growth (and loss of hair on the temples, sometimes it triggers male pattern baldness which is irreversible even if you stop using Testosterone or T. Deepening of your voice (This can be like an adolescent boy's voice 'breaking' and you can lose vocal range if you sing). Thickening of your skin and making you more tolerant of cold. Changing your body odour and increasing sweating. Testosterone may cause a small amount of growth if you haven't finished puberty and still have some growth left in your body. Testosterone also stops your menstrual cycle, generally within 3 months (depending on your dose). Your sex drive will likely increase, as will your appetite. Your clitoris will also begin to grow. The clitoris and penis develop from the same cells in the fetal stage, and T triggers its enlargement. Usually it grows to become 2-5cm (about 1-2 inches). The size will vary between flaccid and erect states like a cis-male's. This is important for metoidioplasty (one of the two options for bottom surgery), which uses the enlarged clitoris to form the penis. Beginning hormone therapy is very much like going through a second puberty; note that if you had acne the first time around, you may once again develop acne, or your skin may become more oily. There is no exact time frame for physical changes, but your menstrual cycle should cease within 6 months. Your voice will likely be at its deepest around after 6 months to a year, the same is true regarding clitoral growth.

Wikipedia Contributors. "Transgender Hormone Therapy (Female-to-Male)." Wikipedia, Wikimedia Foundation, 16 May 2019,en.wikipedia.org/wiki/Transgender_hormone_therapy_(female-to-male). Accessed 24 Apr. 2020.

Chapter Ten

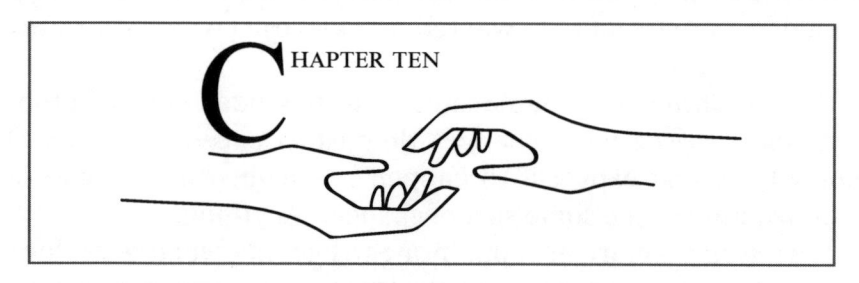

Shay's Journey

My next appointment at the clinic was three months later, in November 2014. Julie and I continued to attend every appointment together. I was looking forward to this appointment and hoped the doctor would refer me for top surgery. I had tried hard to lose weight, working out with a personal trainer twice a week, so I was feeling very positive. As I walked in, the doctor remarked that I was masculinising well and that my arms and shoulders were changing shape. I hadn't really noticed, to be honest, apart from my nether regions becoming slightly bigger and my libido increasing. I did have a bit more chin stubble, too. The doctor went on to say that my hair line was starting to recede. I laughed - Really? I didn't think so. That is my hair gel, I replied. It had only been three months since starting the testosterone and I think he was just trying to make me feel good about myself.

"Please can I be put forward for my double mastectomy? I want this female chest gone," I said.

"We don't rush into this lightly, but I know you are pushing for it." He asked me to get on the scales, and told me I had put on 2kg since my last medical. I could have cried; I had tried so hard! I had spent time at the gym and was eating better. He reckoned the reason could be the change in hormones, as this was likely to cause muscle gain. As I had now put on weight, my BMI was on the limit for an operation. He wanted it to be 30 or less before he put me forward for surgery. He set me a goal: I needed to lose

12kg before my next appointment, in two months. If I did this he would put me forward for my long-awaited surgery. 12kg sounded an awful lot but I wanted to achieve it. I would give it my best.

I went onto social media sites to watch video clips of other transmen, to see what changes they experienced and when. I knew I couldn't expect it to happen overnight, but I could not help wanting to see some sort of change... Anything.

Two weeks before my appointment, I got my blood tests done so I could take the results with me. The tests show how hormone levels are being sustained throughout the three months. If testosterone levels drop, the amount administered can be adjusted accordingly. We arrived at the clinic and were called through. I had my fingers crossed as he weighed me; I knew I had lost quite a bit, but I wasn't sure if it was enough to be considered for surgery. I had lost a stone(6.35kg): "Is that enough? Please can I have surgery now? I am getting a hairy chest and it's not a good look when you still have a feminine bust." The doctor worked out my BMI. "30.9," he said. "Okay, I will refer you. Just lose some more before your referral comes through."

The smile on my face was massive, I was overwhelmed and excited all at the same time – and so happy.

Chapter Eleven

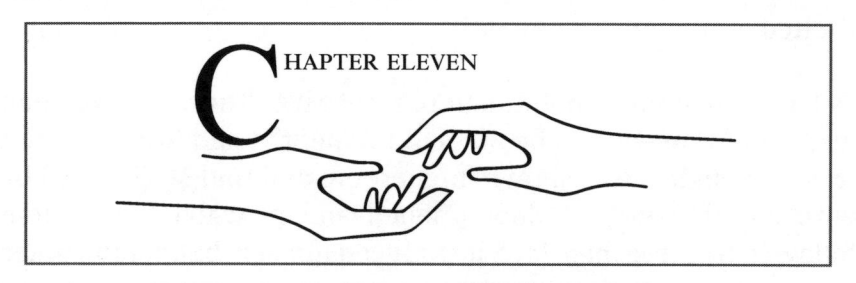

Ready and Waiting

All I could think about was 'when will the letter arrive?' I hoped and prayed that the doctor had sent my referral, and that it didn't get lost in the post. Things had been put back so many times, now I had the go ahead I wanted it to happen there and then. Waiting, when you are told you can have something, seems to drag on forever. I can understand now though, why there is a built-in delay, this is a life changing operation and not something to jump straight into.

During this waiting time things had changed slightly, I had more hair on my chest, arms, thighs and lower legs; but my voice had not deepened. I have been told this is more difficult for the older person transitioning than it is for a teenager - my voice would need to be trained, as it had been as it was for forty years. It was very hard standing in a bank queue with a hairy face, bank card saying Mr on it but having a very heavy chest and a counter attendant asking me if it was my husband's bank card. Embarrassing and not nice, but as you must change your name and all your documents and live in your new chosen gender for two years prior to surgery it is an awkward two years.

Time ticked by and I had not received a letter from the surgery. My three monthly appointment was due on 24th February 2015. On January 12th 2015, a letter from Kettering General Hospital dropped on my mat:

BREAST RECONSTRUCTION APPOINTMENT FEB 4TH 2015
10.30AM
Excited is an understatement!

I arrived at my appointment to meet Mr S. The nurse weighed me, my BMI needed to be 30; had I done it? I had lost 10kg, but was it enough? I was shown into a room and told Mr S would be with me shortly. The door opened and in walked the nurse followed by three men. Mr S introduced himself, but not the other men. I was a bit taken aback to be honest, and felt like a guinea pig being stared at. After a while, I asked who the men were and was told they were trainee plastic surgeons who might attend my surgery. After a brief discussion about my period of transitioning, Mr S asked me to go behind a curtain and remove my top. I don't know why I bothered with the curtain, because everyone looked in on me, which felt uncomfortable. He examined my chest and took some measurements, then drew diagrams to show how the operation would happen and what sort of surgery he thought would suit me best - there are different methods according to the size of chest you currently have. In my case, Mr S recommended the double incision / bilateral method, which involves detaching the whole nipple and re-stitching it in the correct place. Mr S explained everything in detail, including possible complications.

Double incision/Bilateral mastectomy
For individuals with a medium to large breast, horizontal incisions are made to breasts, and mammary glands and fatty tissue are removed. Chest muscles are not touched. Excess chest skin is trimmed, and the incisions closed, leaving scars below the pectoral muscles. Usually, nipples are removed, trimmed, and grafted onto the chest. Alternatively, a "pedicle" technique is used, where nipples are left partially attached to the body, then repositioned and perhaps trimmed. This may maintain sensation in the nipples. If nipples cannot be retained or nipple grafts are lost to tissue death, nipples may be tattooed on later.

Before the incisions are sealed, "drains" are placed along their length. Tubing exits the body through an incision under each armpit, and is attached to a plastic bulb on either side to drain and collect excess blood/fluid. Drains remain in place for several days and need to be emptied. Surgery takes 3 to 4 hours, under general anaesthesia, usually on an outpatient basis. Drains and sutures are removed at post-surgical visits, and healing progress is checked. A binder is worn to aid healing.

Two weeks off work usually allows for healing. If moderate or heavy lifting, or raising arms above the head, is involved, a month or two away is required to avoid risk of scarring and complications. This surgery usually leads to a well-contoured male chest, with two horizontal or U-shaped scars below the pectoral area. Muscle development and chest hair growth can make scars less noticeable. Proper repositioning and resizing of nipples makes for a male-looking chest. There will be partial or complete loss of nipple sensation, and potential loss of nipple grafts due to tissue death. Nipple size, appearance or placement might not be pleasing. There may be excess, protruding skin at the end of the incision or puckering along the scars. Numbness in the armpits due to liposuction, and the usual risks of any surgery, including bleeding, infection, problems from anaesthesia, blood clots, or death (rare).

Keyhole/Peri-areolar incision
For individuals with small amounts of breast tissue, both techniques are done via incisions around the areola (the area of darker skin around the nipple), though the techniques differ. In the keyhole method, a small incision is made along the border of the areola (usually along the bottom), and the breast tissue is removed via liposuction needle. The nipple is left attached to the body via a pedicle (a stalk of tissue) to maintain sensation. Once the breast tissue has been removed, the incision is closed. The nipple is usually not resized or repositioned. In the peri-areolar method, an incision is made along the entire circumference of the areola. The nipple is usually left attached to the body via a pedicle to maintain sensation.

Breast tissue is then "scooped out" by scalpel, or with a combination of scalpel and liposuction. The areola may be trimmed somewhat to reduce its size. Excess skin on the chest may also be trimmed away along the circumference of the incision. The skin is then pulled taut toward the centre of the opening and the nipple is reattached to cover the opening. The nipple/areola may be repositioned, depending on original chest size and the available skin. Excess blood and fluid are drained off by insertion of drain tubes through the original incision and along the pectoral area, exiting the body under the armpits. The tubing is attached to a small plastic bulb on either side, which are left in place for several days. Drains need to be periodically emptied of fluid.

The surgery takes 3 to 4 hours, under general anaesthesia, usually on an outpatient basis. Drains and sutures and removed at post-operative visits, when overall healing progress. A binder is usually worn to aid healing. The surgery does not leave significant visible scarring and usually allows retention of sensation in the nipples. Nipple placement may not be ideal, the chest may not appear completely flat, there is risk of nipple loss due to liposuction trauma of surrounding tissue and numbness from liposuction there may be sagging or puckering.

It was up to me to make the choice, but as Mr S considered the first option the best for me, I decided to go with what he suggested. He checked my weight and told me I needed to lose even more before the surgery could happen. I was disappointed; I had lost over 10kg: nearly 1.5 stone. He explained that he couldn't give me an 18-year-old chest with a 40-year-old belly! Okay, I could understand his point. He gave me two months to lose more weight and tone up, and said he would match my chest to my, hopefully, flatter stomach. The last thing I wanted was moobs! I left the hospital, determined.

In the meantime, I had another appointment with Dr T, at my gender clinic. I was masculinising well as always. From my blood results he saw the testosterone I was taking (testogel) seemed to be changing into oestrogen, which can happen sometimes.

He suggested I switch to Nebido, which involves a three-monthly injection instead of a daily gel. This could be coincided with my three monthly prostap injection. I thought this was a great idea; although I always hated injections, I was getting used to them. This would make things so much more real; taking away the everyday reminder of rubbing in gel. Dr T would write to my GP to change the prescription. Back at my GP's, I asked him if he could issue the prescription straight away, as I had recently had the prostap, and would like the two treatments to coincide. Sure enough, the GP issued the prescription and I came back the following day to see the nurse.

Nebido is an oily drug, so it must be injected slowly over a minute or two, directly into the muscle at the top of the buttock. Boy, did this hurt! All I kept thinking was: it is once every three months; I can do this. I left the surgery happy I would not have to use the gel anymore, so I could forget about everything for the next three months. Walking to the car hurt and when I got in the car I found it very painful to sit on the injected area. I searched the internet during the next few days as the injected area remained very painful and I was unsure whether this was to be expected. I didn't want to be a wuss, but I didn't have anyone to ask.

The injection site was now swollen, hard, hot, red, itchy, and increasingly painful. The internet indicated the injection can be painful and I didn't want to be over dramatic. I waited about a week for it to improve, it didn't, so I called my clinic, to be told there were no consultants available for a week due to annual leave. I eventually called Charing Cross Hospital, London. I had never been there, but just hoped someone could reassure me. I am still awaiting their call-back! I decided to go to A&E. A doctor there asked me why I was taking testosterone, and who had given me the injection. He was quite rude and didn't have a clue how to treat my problem. After briefly visually examining the area, which was like an oversized hot tennis ball in my buttock, his diagnosis was that I had a localised reaction to the drug. He gave me antibiotics and told me to see my own GP in seven days.

Over the next few days the pain grew worse - I was struggling to sit down and even to walk. I called in to see the nurse at the GP surgery; she took one look at my buttock and said it wasn't right. She touched the area and when she felt how hot and hard the area was she went to fetch the GP. The doctor examined the area and prescribed antihistamines and hydrocortisone cream. He suggested that the area might have become infected and advised me to get back in touch with the gender clinic. A week later I emailed the clinic with a brief description and some pictures of my buttock. I got a reply saying my email had been relayed to a consultant who would be in touch shortly. I started to think that I should go back to using the gel as I wouldn't be able to cope with this pain again. The clinic contacted me with an appointment and four days later I arrived to see my consultant. As soon as he saw my buttock, he said I had a haematoma, a very large one at that, and that the injection should have been given an inch higher up. The doctor insisted I get my GP to do an ultrasound scan on the area asap, to confirm his diagnosis. I received a letter from the ultrasound company within three days of the scan, confirming the presence of fluid within the muscle tissue, but not whether it had been a haematoma. It had started to disperse into the body by that point, and eventually the pain went away. It was only six weeks until the injection was due again; I was very on edge about that, but decided to give it another go, as being on gel for the rest of my life was not appealing!

Chapter Twelve

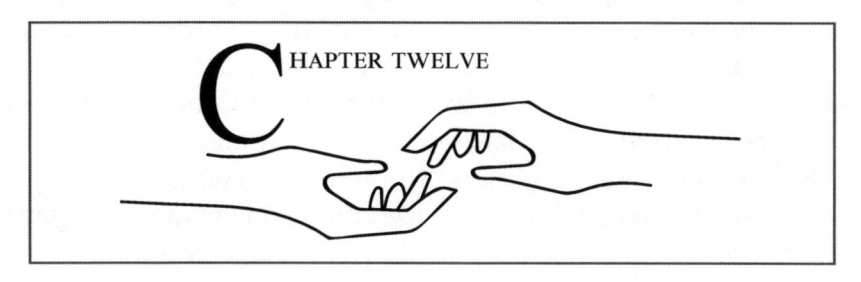

Top Surgery

In May 2015, I had another appointment with Dr S to see how I was progressing. I was very excited! Could this be it? It was! The surgeon was very pleased with my weight loss and agreed to go ahead and give me a date. I felt overwhelmed; obviously this was something I had wanted for a long time, and I was looking at him searching in his diary for a date for me to have my surgery. How did I feel about June 15th? he asked. "Yes, please!" I said, without hesitation. Dr S put my name in his diary and told me I would receive a letter of confirmation. I left the hospital ecstatic. My top surgery was happening; I had waited a life time for this and it was only a month away.

    I know people struggle with work commitments and can't just take dates at short notice, but I am lucky enough to be able to accept dates whenever they are given. Within a few days that confirmation letter hit my mat and I read it so many times I lost count.

KETTERING HOSPITAL SURGERY DATE 15TH JUNE 2015 07.30AM

As the time got nearer I knew I needed to tell my dad. He had no idea I had been on treatment for the last couple of years. He had looked past the fact I now had stubble, and as he never asked, and I didn't know how to approach the subject, we continued to work together every day and I guess he just didn't notice. Now, I needed to tell him, as I wouldn't be at work for a while. The last thing I wanted to do was upset him, and I just didn't know what to expect. When we went on a weekend caravan trip with Dad and my brother, about two weeks prior to my surgery date, I knew time was creeping up on me. He was sitting in our caravan when I turned to him and said: "Dad, what are you doing on June 15th?" He looked in his diary and said, "Not too much, why?"

"I'm going into hospital for an operation and I won't be at work for a few weeks."

"Why, what's wrong?" he asked.

"Nothing is wrong, Dad; I am having my chest removed. I don't like it; I have never liked it. I don't want to be a woman; I want to be a man." His next words shook me:

"Do what whatever makes you happy, as long as you are telling me the truth and you're not ill." I needn't have worried! He made a note of the hospital date in his diary, and told us he would keep the business open as well as he could, and be there for us. I looked at Julie and wondered if it had actually sunk in, but he really wasn't fazed at all.

It was the morning of June 15th, 2015. I hadn't slept much at all, not through worry, because this was something I had been dreaming of for so long, but because I had so little idea of what would actually happen on the day. We arrived at the hospital at 7.15am, and waited in reception. It wasn't long before we were called through, and went up one floor with quite a lot of other people who were there for various types of day surgery. I gave my name, but they couldn't find it on the list, I handed over my letter and they asked me to wait a minute, then came back to me and apologised - the reception nurse had sent me to the wrong place. I would be staying for one or two nights, depending on recovery time.

I found the floor I was supposed to be on and they welcomed me in. They were very friendly. A nurse took me to my room - I had been told I would be on a male ward, and there was a male sign on my door. However, the nurse must have seen my chest, and obviously didn't know what I was there for, so changed the sign to 'female'. The ward sister came over and told her to turn it back.

I was due to have a double incision with nipple grafts, as prior to surgery I was quite big-chested (38FF) and this surgery was more suited to bigger chests. I was in my room for about an hour before a nurse came in and asked me to put on a gown and socks, and said that the consultant would be up shortly to talk with me. She took my blood pressure, then left, and it was another hour before the consultant came to see me. He told me I was third on his surgery list, so I should be going down to theatre at around 11am. He got out his permanent marker pen and proceeded to draw on me. There were a lot of lines and I couldn't understand where he would be starting and finishing. He asked if I had any questions, reassured me everything would be completely fine, and said he would see me shortly.

Time was ticking away, the waiting made me nervous but very excited at the same time. A nurse walked in: "Shay, we are ready for you now."

I walked down to theatre with Julie and the nurse and sat down outside. It was 11.15am. Whilst sitting there I had the thought that nobody had weighed me. The doctors had made such a thing about my weight and now they hadn't even checked it. I was intrigued to know my current weight - I had tried so hard. The first time I went to see the consultant I had weighed 15st 2lb, the last time I saw Dr S I had been 12st 7lb and my BMI was 30.4. I asked the nurse to bring over the scales: my new weight was 11st 4lb - I was well impressed and felt good too.

The door opened and I was called in. It was 11.45am. There were five or six people in a room full of machinery. It was a scary environment, but the people were very friendly – asking me questions to help me feel at ease. They asked me to lie on the bed. I can remember them putting a cannula in the back of my hand, flushing through with saline, then injecting the anaesthetic. The next thing I remember is waking up in the recovery room. I was told I had been in theatre for 3.5 hours. They wheeled me back to my room where it was lovely to find Julie waiting for me. I couldn't see my chest as I had a large waterproof covering stuck to me.

I was awake but a bit hazy that afternoon. I can remember the evening though. They were checking my blood pressure every hour as it was really low, I also know that at 7.30pm the nurse looked at my cannula and said it wasn't working. It was really hurting the back of my hand. She took it out, said she would get someone to put another one in as I needed my antibiotics intravenously, and someone would be with me shortly. Julie left me at 9pm and, despite us reminding them, the cannula still wasn't in place. I was very tired, but didn't want to go to sleep to be woken back up by someone wanting to replace the cannula, so tried my hardest to stay awake. I texted Julie at midnight to tell her they still hadn't put it in - I was worried because I needed those antibiotics regularly. The nurse came in at 12.30am to put my antibiotics into a cannula that still wasn't in place. She said she would go and get someone. A nurse came in about ten minutes later, looked at my hands and said my veins weren't good. "I will get the doctor to do it," she said. The doctor finally came in at 1am and instead of putting it into the back of my hand she finally inserted the cannula just inside my right elbow. Fifteen minutes later I had my antibiotics, I could now go to sleep - so I thought.

fifteen minutes later, the nurse came to take my blood pressure. I was half asleep when she put the cuff monitor on over the new cannula. As pressure was applied, I thought the needle was going to fly out of my arm. Boy, did that hurt. Once I winced, the nurse realised what she had done, took it off and put it onto the other arm. My blood pressure was still low, but at least I could sleep.

I woke up early for breakfast, then at 9.30am Julie arrived to see me. At 10am the nurse came in to remove my drains, which was slightly uncomfortable but not too painful. At 11am the nurse told me I didn't have to wait and see the consultant, once my medication arrived I would be free to go. I must admit I would rather have seen the surgeon, just for a bit of explanation really. A different nurse brought in my painkillers and antibiotics. So did that mean I could leave? I dressed with Julie's help, and packed my bag, then I couldn't find a nurse so we left. It seemed really strange as I had expected some kind of discharge, but there was nothing at all. I felt very happy and very dozy. My smile was immense, and the pain wasn't too bad. I would have to go back in one week for them to check the wounds and remove the waterproof dressing. I would find out, then, if my nipple grafts had taken, as sometimes the graft can die - something that played on my mind all week.

Chapter Thirteen

The Big Reveal and Further Surgery

I arrived the following week, for the big reveal, scared, excited, all emotions running wild. This was the first time I would see my chest and nipples after my surgery. What would I actually look like? I met with a nurse I had seen once before. When I was ready, the waterproof coating, which was more like a massive piece of very sticky tape stuck right across me, was peeled back. I was trying my hardest to watch, and so was Julie; it seemed an eternity as we watched every inch peel off. I looked down and was speechless, I just stared in amazement: it was great. My chest was obviously still swollen, but I was so impressed. Both my nipple grafts had taken, so no worry there. And here was the chest I had craved. I can't thank that surgeon enough for lifting my soul and giving me a chest that looks so great. Happy is an understatement. I now had to be careful, take my time, no heavy lifting, and return for a review in eight weeks. What a difference I could already see in myself. My confidence soared and I felt much better. I was back at work within two weeks. I have a physical job so had to be careful, but Julie came to work and helped me do things until I was back on my feet properly. People commented on how well I looked, which was all down to the new body I had and how it made me feel. Lots of bio oil rubbed into my scars eased the tightness, I healed well and within six months I was looking at chest tattoo designs.

67

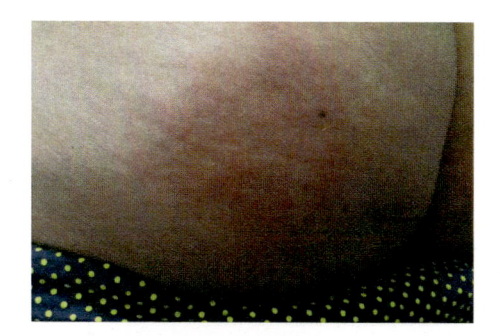

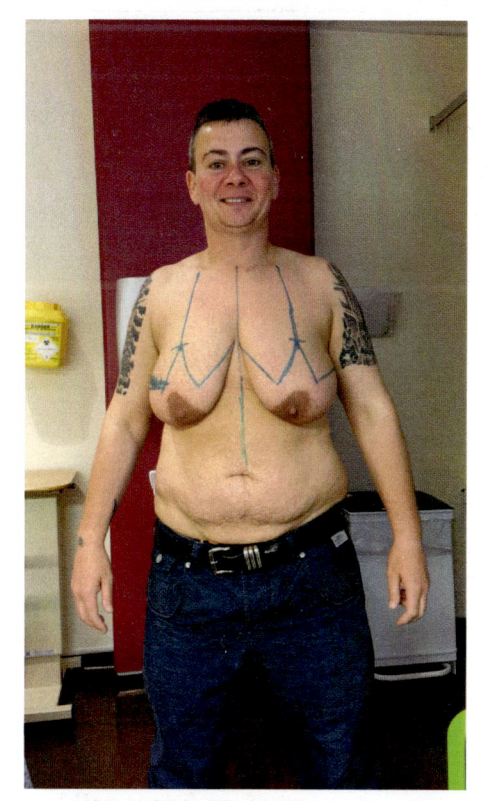

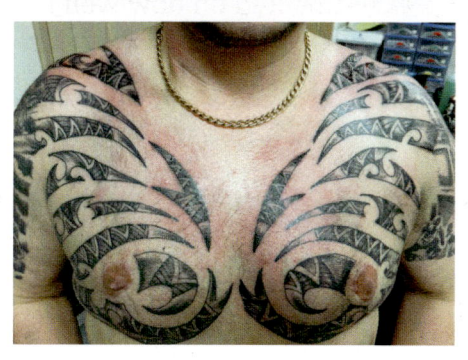

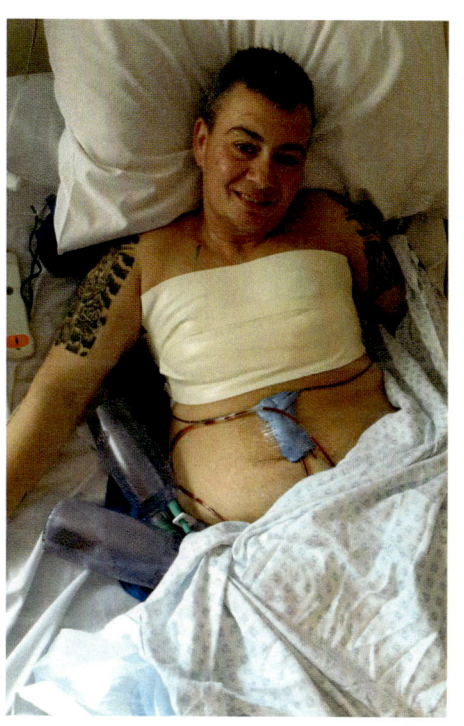

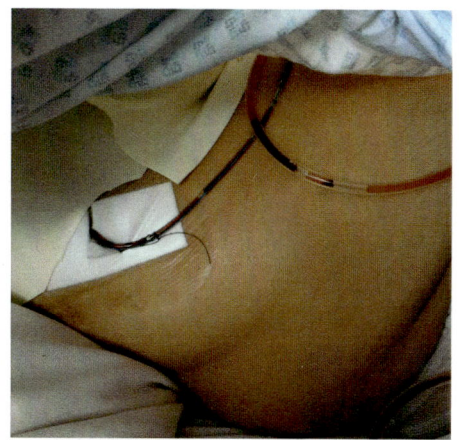

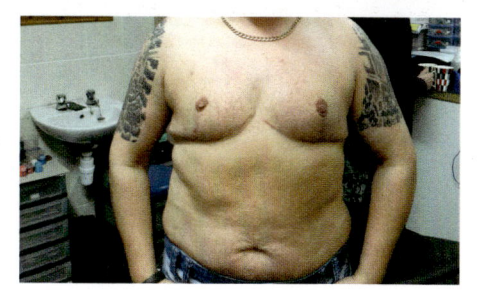

I searched the internet for tattoos, mainly because I now felt self-conscious about my scar lines. They were not bad, but were under each of the old breasts. I didn't want any trace of femininity to remain, and never wanted to be asked why I had scars. I wanted a completely male chest. In time, I found a tattooist who looked at my chest and said, as I had healed so well, he would tattoo me. I found a few designs I liked then let him come up with something for me. I had to have three sittings in total, as the pain was quite harsh in certain areas and over some of the scar lines, but each sitting made me feel better and better. I had decided on a tribal tattoo, as I found this masculine and we could incorporate both my scars. The result is, I love it.

Probably a week or two after my tattoo, I received a letter from St.Peter's Andrology centre giving me an appointment to see a surgeon regarding my lower surgery. I was excited at how quickly things were moving for me. My appointment was in January 2016. I met the surgeon - Dr G. He was lovely, and really thorough, explaining things well, showing me diagrams of how things would look and work. He told me there were several options and I must be fully sure about them all and which route I would like to take. The options available were:

- HYSTERECTOMY (removal of the uterus – womb)

- SALPINGO-OOPHORECTOMY (removal of the fallopian tubes and ovaries)

- VAGINECTOMY (removal of the vagina)

- METOIDIOPLASTY (creates a micro-penis by bringing the clitoris forward)

- URETHROPLASTY (creates a repositioned, longer urethra – the tube you urinate through. This is joined to your existing urethra – the "hook-up")

- PHALLOPLASTY (creates a penis)

- SCROTOPLASTY (creates a scrotum and generally includes testicular prostheses, often a later stage)

- ERECTILE IMPLANTS (creates erectile capability)

Obviously, there is a lot to consider. The removal of the uterus and ovaries makes you infertile, so it is an important decision, but I already had two of my own children and two step children and we didn't want any more. There are serious risks involved, significant bleeding, damage to bowel and/or bladder and/or urethra, pulmonary embolism, deep vein thrombosis, anaesthetic problems, wound breakdown and infection. These were the risks associated with just the first part of the total hysterectomy. But still, knowing all of this, I wanted to go ahead.

The first stage for me was going to be a hysterectomy, so I lay on the couch and the doctor examined my stomach. He said I had excess skin – not surprising having had two children, I felt I had a massive spare tyre. Jokingly, I asked if I could have a tummy tuck. His response was to recommend one. Oh yes, I thought, I'm going to have a six pack. The skin needed to be lifted so the phallus could be attached without being too low. I decided I wanted the full works, the hysterectomy, bilateral salpingo-oophorectomy, vaginectomy, phalloplasty, scrotoplasty and erectile implants. This would be over four operations, with a minimum gap of three months to allow time for healing. Dr. G looked in his diary and gave me a date for the total hysterectomy, bilateral salpingo-oophorectomy and tummy tuck, all at the same time - Friday 4th March 2016. Could I make that date? Oh yes, I could make it. My appointment was going to be at Highgate Hospital in London. I was so excited. The weeks couldn't pass quickly enough.

We checked in at Highgate at 6pm on Friday 4th March. My operation was on the Saturday morning, I didn't know what time. I signed in and was asked what newspaper I would like. Wow, I didn't expect that. My room was very nice; there was a telephone next to my bed so if I wanted anything - sandwich, coffee, ice cream, cooked meal - I could pick up the phone and it was brought up to the room by a man in a waistcoat who looked like a butler and carried a sliver tray. It was more of a hotel than a hospital: I felt very spoilt. The staff were amazing; even before my operation, they would come to talk to me and to ask if I wanted anything. I recommend this hospital!

I settled in, and Julie stayed with me until 9.30pm, then she left for the hotel we had booked her into. When she left, my nerves started to kick in. I knew this was what I wanted, but I was also nervous of the operating table. I didn't sleep much that night, but 7am came around quite quickly and before I knew it, Julie was back. We didn't know what time my operation was to be, but there are no formal visiting times and she was allowed in. Everyone was happy to help.

The surgeon came to see me at around 8am and said I would be going down second, which should be around 11am. He went through all the paperwork with me, explaining everything again, and I signed some consent forms. He told me what would happen in surgery and said I should be there for about three hours. He told me I would be staying in hospital for about three days if everything went well. He asked if there was anything I needed to know, but I felt completely that I was in the right hands. He told me he would see me in theatre and that the anaesthetist would be with me shortly.

About thirty minutes later the anaesthetist came to see me again, went through my notes, introduced himself and explained what he would be doing and that he would be with me the whole time. Once I start to come around I would be taken to recovery and then back up to my room. Asked if there was anything I didn't understand, I said I was fully aware of what was happening. They gave me plenty of chances to ask questions and clarify things.

Within twenty-five minutes the nurse came to take me down to theatre. I had on the gown and slippers provided, and Julie and I were taken to the lift, at which point Julie was not allowed any further. She gave me the biggest hug and told me she would be waiting for me. I was taken down the cleanest corridor I had ever seen: it was sparkling white, not a mark anywhere, then into a room with a bed, where I was to meet the anaesthetist. I sat on the couch and the staff were all laughing and joking with me, telling me what a nice man the anaesthetist was. He put a cannula into my hand and washed it through with saline solution, which was cold and a bit stingy. He explained that in a minute he would be putting in the anaesthetic and I would just drift off to sleep. He asked me to lie down and was talking to me, but I cannot remember any more...

I woke up in the recovery area, still dozy, and was taken back up to my room, where my beloved was waiting for me. Julie had been panicking as they had told us surgery would take about three hours, but I was away for just over five hours including recovery time. She began to think something had happened to me, but as my blood pressure was low they kept me longer. I had the tummy tuck as well, so this extended the surgery time. I cannot remember too much that day, apart from nurses checking my blood pressure every half hour at first, then every hour. I can remember drifting in and out and them bringing me some food, which I really didn't feel like eating, but the ice cream was good. I have to say I didn't really feel any pain, with pain killers administered every four hours, I just felt tired. When the nurses passed the room they would stick their head in and ask if I wanted anything. Cup of tea? I liked it there and felt very looked after. Nothing was too much trouble, day or night.

Later in the day, I felt more myself and actually pulled back the covers to have a look at what had been done. There was nothing much to see apart from a couple of drains and a lot of dressings across my middle. They had applied a catheter, so no need to get out and go to the toilet, which I was relieved about. Even though I didn't have a lot of pain when lying in my bed, I needed help to sit up. I had been told there were fifty-six staples across my stomach, which seemed massive. I hadn't realised I was being stapled, I just presumed I would be stitched, but I didn't know how big my incision line would be. I was feeling on top of the world in myself.

Julie had stayed with me until the ward shut at 9.30pm. She left to go back to her room and I just wanted to sleep. All through the night, though, I was monitored closely, with the nurses coming in regularly, as my blood pressure remained low. Having the blood pressure cuff and pressure cuffs on each leg to aid circulation inflating every five or ten minutes, disturbed my sleep.

I actually fancied my breakfast next morning: fruit juice, yogurt, toast, scrambled egg, tomato, bacon, beans - I enjoyed it. Julie arrived after breakfast and the nurses were in with me checking my drains and about to remove and change the dressings. I hadn't drained a lot of blood, which apparently is a good sign as things are healing well. They suggested I might get my drains removed that day. They started to remove my dressings and to be honest I really wasn't sure what I would be looking at. I knew what surgery I had gone in for and prior to this I had searched the internet for pictures of operations, but there were so many out there, scary ones at that, that I stopped looking. Also, this wasn't just a hysterectomy; it was the tummy tuck as well. Once the dressings were removed I was staring at a swollen stomach with a very neat incision line which went all the way across. There was a 'nipple' at each end, where they had tied off; that was the only bit I was unsure about. They told me not to worry as at the next stage they could take off the excess skin and use it somewhere else. It was stunning work.

That afternoon, my drains were removed and I was due to get up. I was worried about this, as sitting up felt very awkward and uncomfortable. I was still on a high dose of pain killers but felt very weak. The nurse came back and said "Come on then, you're getting up and going in the shower." I looked at Julie and wondered if I could actually do this. However, I am not one to give up on anything and will try my absolute hardest in everything I do. The bed was lowered enough for me to be able to get out.

The nurses were still concerned about my low blood pressure, so asked me to take deep breaths. To my surprise, with a nurse at either side, I stood up, and with each step I took I smiled. I was taken to the shower cubicle and they helped me take off my gown, put everything within my reach and turned on the shower. That was a lovely feeling, to be nice and clean.

Instead of getting back into bed, I sat in my chair for the afternoon. I felt so much better. I was still on regular pain medication, but felt good. My dinner arrived, and they brought Julie some dinner too. Soup to start, lamb shank, mash and vegetables, followed by Haagen Daz ice cream, very nice. The afternoon passed and my blood pressure improved. They kept telling me to drink plenty of water. Evening came and Julie went back to her room, I would be going home the next day. I was excited to go home and slightly nervous too, as we have four cats that like to jump on the bed and I was worrying about how we could stop them from jumping or lying on me.

I woke to the nurse bringing in my meds and checking my obs, very lovely staff, always making me smile. I was so pleased to have met them and with the care they gave me whilst I was there. The consultant/surgeon came to see me and said he was happy with how the operation went, I was healing really well and I was all good to go home once they had organised my medication. I shook his hand and thanked him so much; I liked Dr G, he was pleasant and made me feel comfortable enough to ask him anything. The nurse bought in my medication and discharge note and said they would contact my GP with details of the care I needed, and that I would need my staples taken out in fourteen days, which would be arranged for me. We packed up my stuff, well Julie did, said our goodbyes and I was wheeled in a chair down to the front door of the reception area. Julie bought up the car to the door and I walked to my car.

Getting in the car was a struggle and the two hour journey home, sitting in the same position, was uncomfortable. We managed it, though, even getting my latte on the way home. I was happy to be in my home surroundings, with my animals and Julie - now my full time carer. I sat on the settee and watched television for an hour, then decided I wanted to lie down for a while so went upstairs. After twenty minutes I had all four cats on the bed, trying to lie on me. Whilst I would normally like this, I couldn't move quick enough to push them off and one jumped from the floor onto me, making me cry in pain. It wasn't their fault, they didn't know, they just wanted to see me. Julie came rushing up, gave me some more painkillers then disappeared for a while, returning with a present she had made me. It was a kind of cage, made of cardboard, to stop the cats walking on my stomach and hurting me. Something so simple, but so thoughtful, allowed me to relax and be comfortable, and not worry that if I fell asleep they might jump onto me. We never thought about it until we were home, but I know you can buy bed cages and dinner trays online and this is something to consider getting, especially if you have animals. Julie's invention was so useful, I was very grateful.

For the next couple of days, I could manage going to the toilet and going back to bed but that was just about all. Julie brought me breakfast and cups of tea and I carried on taking my painkillers. I was generally tired and slept a lot. By day three I was doing the stairs: it was difficult, but I wanted to get around. I would come downstairs, watch television and have something to eat, but when I sat for long my stomach felt squashed and uncomfortable, so lying down was easier. Even though I wanted to be up, my body didn't feel ready yet. I would wait for Julie to get home to help me have a shower as our shower was in the bath and trying to lift my leg hurt; I found it easier to sit on the side of the bath and swivel myself in. Getting out was harder still, as trying to put a foot down to the floor without bending too much was awkward. I also wanted her to be around in case I slipped. I normally have a shower every day, so not having one daily because you can't get your dressings wet was out of character for me and made me think I might smell.

Things got gradually easier over the week, and on day seven I even went for a trip up to the local supermarket as a passenger, just because I wanted to get out. I took things slowly and did what I could. One day, Julie took to me to work to see how things were going, and to see work friends. On day nine I started back to work. I am a tyre fitter and couldn't do physical work, but I could answer the phone, deal with questions and take orders.

Day fourteen was when my dressings would be removed completely and the staples taken from my tummy tuck. I can't say I was looking forward to this; as I was no longer on painkillers I thought it was really going to hurt, but in all honesty it didn't. I could feel it pulling, but nothing more. The nurse counted as each one was taken out – fifty six she counted; that's good, I thought, as that's how many they put in.

When the nurse had finished, she said my tummy looked really good and I had healed really well. She advised that it would help the area feel more supple if I rubbed bio oil or E45 cream into my skin daily, and especially into the excess skin at the sides of my abdomen. As I didn't like these nipple type pieces, I paid a lot of attention to that area. They didn't disappear but I was told not to worry, as this would be rectified later. I had expected the tummy tuck to leave my abdomen flat, though obviously swollen, but it looked as though I had big ears on the side of me and a big saggy stomach. As time went on I returned to work full time and started fitting tyres again after about seven weeks. I knew when things were too heavy and didn't strain myself. I was just happy.

I was told by the surgeon that the minimum time between each operation is three months, which gives the body time to heal and return to normal. In that case, the earliest I would be looking at for my next stage would be June. I had said I could be ready at the drop of a hat, as I am one of the lucky ones who does not need to give my employer a lot of notice. I was feeling good in myself. To lose the weight prior to my operations, I had a personal trainer who got me where I needed to be. I wasn't ready to train again, but I did want the look of that belly to disappear. I felt that all the work I had done before the op was going out the window, as I wasn't exercising but was still eating. The weight was creeping back on. Unsure what to do, I started to walk around the block, and soon I was running around, doing a bit more each day.

Chapter Fourteen

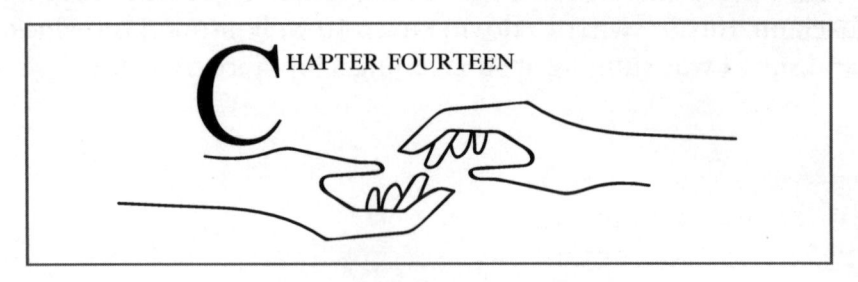

Life Changes - The Biggy

On the morning of Friday, June 10th, I had a phone call from St.Peter's Andrology centre in London, asking if I still wanted a short notice time slot. "Yes!" I said.

"How do you feel about coming in this Sunday for your operation on Monday?" I think gob-smacked was how I felt!

"Errmmm, two days' time?" I said. "Yes, please. Where do I go?"

As it was such short notice there wouldn't be time to send out a letter; he would send me an email with details. I was excited. Julie knew I was on the phone to them and stared at me, waiting for my reaction. I sat down. Two days' time? I wasn't expecting that! I knew I wanted it as fast as possible, but I didn't know whether such short notice was good or bad. Panic hit, as this was the biggest of all operations: life-changing. This was the major Biggy!

I would be in hospital for at least seven days and had nobody to cover my work or care for our animals. I had to pack a bag and find somewhere for Julie to stay for the week, as she was always by my side and would never let me be in hospital on my own. A lot to sort out, but I could do this. I was anxious, happy, excited, scared sick and worried. Normally, Julie answers the phone at work but I do the manual work, I needed to make sure that things were up to date, bills were paid and orders were all set up.

The thing is, we didn't have a lot of money, and definitely couldn't afford to stay in London for a week. Julie said she would sleep in the car, staying in the hospital until 10pm and returning at 7am, but I wasn't happy with her doing that.

That night, I expected us to be happy, cuddling in bed, but we were both upset and scared. We were not financially stable, so we needed the garage to be open. Julie kept crying, which in turn upset me. I tried to explain that this was what I wanted. She understood, but negative thoughts were crossing her mind – what if things went wrong? I was having thoughts about dying on the table, but there was no way I was going to let her know that. I was prepared to put myself through all of this to get the body I wanted, this was not a whim, it was my life I was playing with. It was just the run up to it, I guess. I had waited a long time, but now it was happening it kind of stopped me in my tracks. I wanted it to be a happy moment, but it was more like being on a roller coaster. I made a video before this and every operation, so that if anything happened, my thoughts and feelings were recorded. I was putting on a very brave face, as though I was not bothered at all, but inside I was petrified and my head felt as if it was being squashed in a vice.

Julie said she didn't want to be on her own for around eleven hours, worrying about me down in theatre. I tried to reassure her. She wanted to stay with me all week, but I asked her to keep the business open for us, to which she reluctantly agreed. We decided she would stay with me for a couple of days, return home with a friend, then come back to me later in the week. I would be bedridden for a few days, so it made sense really.

The following morning, 12th June 2016, I put down the seats in my car, put in a quilt and some pillows and then another quilt on top to make up a bed for Julie. I bought her a teddy and tucked it inside, so she would find it that night. We set off to London – not speaking much, emotions running high. We went to see my kids and grandkids, hiding my doubts and the severity of the operation. My youngest wished me luck, whereas I think it just went over the head of my oldest, maybe because this had become day to day life by now. I had good luck wishes from both my aunties, and my friends. Dad knew I was going into hospital, but I was very vague. I was doing what I knew would make me happy, I didn't want to worry them, I would be fine.

During the journey, Julie took a picture of my arm. This was the last time my arm would look as it looked then. After the operation I would have a skin graft taken and the tattoo that was currently on my arm would be gone. It said: "Julie, My Partner, My Love, My Life".

We checked in at the hospital and were shown to my room. I could pick up the phone and order anything I wanted up until 12pm. Nurses checked my blood pressure, took some blood and swabs and gave us paperwork to sign. I was given a diary of what would be happening to me over the next week:

- Return to ward post-surgery: 1 hourly phallus pulse checked, if no pulse apparent, consultant to be contacted immediately, BP to kept above 100 systolic, urine output over 30mls per hour, strict bed rest.
- Day 1 after op: strict bed rest, 1 hourly Dopplers (pulse check in phallus) for 24 hours (Warmth and Capillary refill). Keep phallus elevated at 45 degree angle, arm to remain elevated in Bradford sling for 5 days, fingertip touching and straightening hand only, keep an eye on warmth, sensation, movement and capillary refill. Clean and redress phallus and buttock donor site wounds as needed. Check phallus for any duskiness, particularly on the ventral aspect. Check full blood count, drains and urethral catheter to remain.
- Day 2: strict bed rest, checks go from every 1 to every 2 hours, keep phallus at 45 degree angle, check phallus for any duskiness, particularly on the ventral area, arm to stay elevated in Bradford sling, check warmth, sensation, movement, and capillary refill of fingers, cleanse and redress wounds as needed. Oral antibiotics and oral pain killers as tolerated. Drains, urethral catheter and stent to remain.

- Day 3: chair to bathroom and daily checks, gentle mobilisation, phallus to remain at 45 degrees, keep check on any duskiness on phallus, 4 hourly phallus pulse test, oral antibiotics and pain killers, possible drain removal and catheter - team to review.
- Day 4: general mobilisation today, daily showers, arm to be kept dry by using a plastic bag to cover, phallus to remain at 45 degrees, check phallus for any duskiness, arm to remain in Bradford sling, wound care as needed. 6 hourly phallus pulse test, oral antibiotics and pain relief.
- Day 5: general mobilisation, eight hourly phallus pulse test, daily shower, keep arm dry, wound care as needed, arm can be relaxed out of Bradford sling, patient must not lift, rotate or flex the wrist for three weeks post-surgery. Continue with hand exercises and start straightening the arm, do not knock the arm as this can damage the graft and cause necrosis.
- Day 6/7: arm dressing taken off, to be redressed with mepitel, gauze, sofban, and crepe bandage, phallus stent comes out (only if patient can pass urine from a different orifice, i.e catheter), wound care as needed, patient to be discharged home if no major complications. District nurse referral.
- Arm & Buttock sutures out 14 days post op.
- Phallus sutures out 21 days post op.
- Arm to be redressed on a weekly basis with mepitel, gauze, softban, and bandage until dry enough to expose.
- Check up at Harley Street 4-5 weeks.

Some of the nurses didn't know I was transgender, which was a nice feeling. One nurse was shocked to know I was a woman previously and said she was amazed at how good I looked. Things were strained between Julie and me that afternoon, simply because there was so much worry. I could see it in Julie's face, but she still wanted whatever I did, and she was happy I was in a lovely place with nice people. I felt good this was happening, but feared the operating table, as I knew the high risks. I had this terrible thought going through my head that I wouldn't survive, or the operation would go completely wrong. I also feared I would have no sexual feeling at all, as the old bits were going and new bits were arriving, but what if the nerves didn't connect, or the skin died?

My arm would be cut to the size decided by the surgeon, to give me the best Ferrari he could. This would then be made into my phallus and attached in the correct place in my pubic area. Then, I would have full thickness skin grafts taken from both of my buttocks to replace the skin and tissue on my arm. So, I was going to be very sore in several places.

I asked the nurses and the doctor if, when they spoke to me, I could record it, because so much was said that I couldn't take it all in. There are different surgical procedures available. One is a metoidioplasty: this is where taking the testosterone causes the clitoris to increase in size to about the length of a thumb. Part of the ligament that holds the clitoris in place, and some surrounding tissue, is taken away, so the surgeon can create a small phallus from the elongated clitoris. This is not ideal, though, for a sexual relationship. I wanted the phalloplasty: this is where a penis is constructed using donor skin from other areas of the body. Skin can be taken from abdomen, groin/leg, or forearm, and grafted onto the pubic area. The urethra is then lengthened so the patient can urinate through the penis. Erections are usually achieved with either a permanent implanted malleable rod or an implanted pump device. I didn't like the idea of bending a rod into place before sex, so chose the pump device, which seemed the closest to 'the real thing'. There are two tubes that run either side inside the penis, a small rugby shaped ball filled with saline, which sits just inside the abdomen, and a little ball with a tiny notch on it, that sits inside one of the newly created testicles. This is all joined with tubing. You squeeze the ball in the testicle, which allows the saline to travel and fill the two tubes, giving an erection: amazing work.

When you want the erection to go down, you just press the little notch. I did have the option to keep the clitoris, but didn't want to look different or to see 'both bits'. I chose to have the clitoris buried under the skin where it cannot be seen and only I can feel it.

Originally I had thought I didn't want skin for the phallus taken from my arm as my sleeves are always rolled up and I didn't want people looking at my arms and asking what I had done. Having the phallus made from the abdomen sounded ideal cosmetically, but there aren't many nerves, so there wouldn't be much feeling. Due to the hairless, smooth nature of the skin on the underside of the arm, this is generally felt to give good results. The nerves and blood vessels are also harvested with the skin. The main drawback is that it leaves a very large scarred area on the forearm. There is also some risk to overall function and feeling of the arm. The forearm skin is shaped into the new phallus and grafted onto the groin and the nerves and blood vessels are connected. Some surgeons connect the brachial nerve of the forearm to the nerve of the clitoris, with the goal being sensation in the phallus. Blood vessels are taken from the forearm and joined with those in the pelvis to ensure the penis has an adequate blood supply. It is usual to take one artery and two or three veins. Nerves are taken from the arm and joined at the base of the penis. It can take many months, maybe up to a year, before the nerves function again, and during this time there will be no sensation in the penis. It is important to be careful not to damage the penis whilst there is no feeling in it. Sometimes sensation can be lost if the nerves don't take, so it is a gamble. The urethra is made using tissue from the labia, inside of the mouth/cheeks, the vaginal wall or with a selection of hairless skin, shaped into an inverted tube and placed inside the phallus. My arm would need a full thickness graft, taken from my buttocks. It would be covered with a pressure garment from six months to a year. I would be called back in for further procedures, as time is needed for healing. At this first stage I would have a phallus but I would still be urinating through my old bits. I would have a vagina and a phallus, but the phallus would have a catheter inside it for a while, allowing the inside of it to heal so I wouldn't be able to urinate through it yet. I was told about possible complications:

- Loss of phallus
- Loss of forearm graft
- Small areas of tissue can die, in rare cases the phallus can be lost
- Urethral stricture
- Urethral fistula

It was very serious stuff I wanted to go for. The way I saw it, once on the operating table, I wanted the whole works. Others have different views depending on their bodies and how they feel.

So, that afternoon was a mixture of worry and happiness. We were made to feel very welcome. I was advised to relax and told my operation would be early the next morning, after seeing the consultant. Bloods were taken, which, to be honest, was very painful. Two days before, I had a tattoo done on the inside of my left arm, from where you would normally take blood, as I hadn't known I was going in for surgery. Of course, the tattoo was sore and fresh, and as you are not allowed any needles in the donor arm, the bloods had to come from my left arm. They couldn't find a vein inside the elbow, so took the blood from the outside, which made me queasy. We chatted all afternoon, with nurses and the consultant coming in to fill forms and make sure I understood what was going to happen and the risks involved. At 8.30pm they wanted me to have a meal, as I wouldn't be eating past midnight. I chose vegetable soup to start, steak, potatoes and vegetables, with Haagen Dazs ice cream. Not the hospital food people would normally expect. I was told I would be going into surgery at 8am the next day but Dr. G would be round earlier.

Online, people talk about between nine and eleven hours surgery, so that kind of puts scary thoughts in your head. One of the nurses told us it would only take four hours, which brought a bit of relief. I now know that she got mixed up, but only found this out afterwards, so Julie was expecting me back after four to five hours. At the time of my hysterectomy, I was told my blood pressure dropped so low that it put me into a coma; this was playing on my mind. Would I survive the table this time? I was apprehensive. Julie had made me a small photo album, which I had next to my bed, I also had a teddy she had bought me before my first operation, to which she attached a St. Christopher to keep me safe. There was a picture of the two of us on the bottom of the bed so I would see us when I came round. At about 10pm, it was time for Julie to go. The nurses gave me sleeping tablets because they wanted me to be rested for the next day, and Julie went to her double bed in the back of the car. We video chatted for a while, then said goodnight. I made a little video on my phone, about how I was feeling: just a few hours left until I got my own willy. I was in a happy mood, relaxed and confident, and looking forward to the next twenty-four hours.

I woke up around 6am with my blood pressure being taken, ready for the big day. I hadn't slept too well, tossing and turning and a bit uncomfortable. My blood pressure was good, at 119/75. Two hours before surgery the nurse came in and said I was to get up, take off my jewellery and have a shower, then she would be back to get me into my gown. The room was warm; I knew I was going to be very sore for a while; I wanted a cup of tea but was not allowed anything; I was nervous, but that was to be expected. I made a little video for Julie, on my phone, telling her I loved her. Even to this day she hasn't seen it.

Julie arrived at about 7am after a night in the car, bless her! She assured me she had been comfortable and was fine. Breakfast was lovely bacon, eggs, beans, the full works, but I was not allowed to eat so Julie tucked in. The assistant consultant came to talk to us about how the day would pan out. He checked which arm was going to be used and drew a big arrow on the back of my hand. He explained that the buttocks graft would be done first, and this would leave a linear scar, which wouldn't be too noticeable. Whilst Dr. G worked on my arm, creating the phallus, Dr. M would be working on my abdomen, preparing and looking for the peripheral and ilioinguinal nerves, arteries and veins, that would be joined together, once the phallus was created, to give sensation and vitality. This would leave a three-inch abdomen scar. He told me about the risks of any operation - bleeding, haematoma, clot formation inside the artery, which could result in total or partial loss of the phallus, which would have to be removed to avoid infection and sepsis. To be told I could lose the phallus was very scary. I asked how many of these procedures take place and was told it was four or five a week, with patients coming from all over the world. He was a lovely chap; he answered all my questions and made me feel at ease. I had tattoos on my left arm, and was concerned about where they would end up. He explained that they may be visible on the tip of my new penis, but if that bothered me, I could have a tattoo down below to hide anything I didn't like. I would be staying in hospital for around seven days, bed-ridden and not moving at all for the first two or three. He shook my hand, I signed some paperwork, and he said he would see me in about thirty minutes.

The doctor left, we took a couple of pictures of my arm, and I put on my gown. A nurse came in who remembered me from my previous operation, and asked if I minded if a student nurse watched the operation. They brought her in to see me and I asked her if she could video the operation, but this wasn't allowed. She would be standing right next to the surgeon. Time was ticking; it was 9am.

At 9.15am another nurse came to go through the paperwork. She checked my name, date of birth, checked my name band, asked if it was my signature on the form, asked what operation I was having, if I had an arrow on my arm, which arm would be operated on, any allergies, the last time I ate or drank, whether I had jewellery, piercings, contact lenses, hearing aids or metal objects. She checked that I had signed a photography consent form. They certainly make sure you know what you are in there for!

The surgeon drew the area that would be taken away from my arm and made into my new phallus. The anaesthetist came to tell me that he would be with me all the time and not to worry about anything. He had a look at my arms and asked me questions again. He explained they would take the skin grafts first, from my buttocks, so I would be face down for a while and there might be a bit of swelling to my face for twenty-four hours or so. He left my room and within ten minutes a nurse came in and said, "Come on, Shay, they are ready for you." It was 9.40am, and my stomach was churning. I pulled on my dressing gown and slippers and walked with Julie and the nurse down the corridor to the lift. This was as far as Julie could go. We hugged and kissed and I said I would be back soon. I could see she was upset, but I would be fine, I was sure of it. I was nervous as anything, to be honest, but I didn't want to show it. I walked through the cleanest hospital ever, bright white walls with sparkles - lush. I went into a small room where the anaesthetist and his friendly staff asked me to sit on the couch. He explained he was going to give me an epidural, to the spine, and also insert a catheter into my hand, which is where the drugs would be administered. I was so nervous I was talking loads, and the more I talked the more I forgot what was going on around me.

I was still sitting on the couch when the anaesthetist went behind me to do the epidural. He said, "slight scratch" but I remember that scratch bloody hurting. Within seconds they were lying me down, and within minutes I couldn't feel my legs. That was not a nice thing at all. It was scary no longer being in control. I can remember looking all around me as they slid me from one couch to another. Once I was on the surgeon's table, I remember him looking and talking to me and other people looking over me. Then the drug was administered. I can remember telling a lady her face was going blurry, and then I can't remember any more until I woke up in the recovery room, with a nurse calling my name. I remember hearing I was ready to be taken back to my room, but I was so tired I was struggling to keep my eyes open. I can also remember struggling to speak, as I had an oxygen mask on. I told the nurse how sick I felt, and she put an anti-sickness drug into my catheter. I also remember being told my blood pressure was low and I needed to be checked every half an hour; it had dropped so low during surgery that the original seven hours that Julie was expecting had turned into nine hours, as I was being watched in recovery for longer. This caused a lot of panic on Julie's side, as she hadn't realised what was going on. Eventually, she rang the recovery room to check I was back.

A man wheeled me back up to my room. I had had major surgery but I didn't feel any pain, just felt tired and dozy and wanted to sleep. I didn't like the mask one little bit, and wanted to take it off, but I wasn't allowed. They wanted to manage my blood pressure as it was staying really low. I arrived back in my room at 7.05pm. I can remember seeing Julie there and her giving me a kiss, but that whole day is a blur. She videoed me later that night, speaking, but this was just to say my arm was hurting (they gave me extra pain killers, making me even more sleepy) and that my bottom was sore from the stitches. I mentioned that I was looking forward to feeling better, but that all went well. Julie took loads of pictures for me, as I wanted to document everything to do with my transition and couldn't do this whilst I was strapped up. My arm had to stay in the air for the whole hospital stay, to aid circulation, which wasn't the most comfortable experience. I had to have a pillow under my arm, as I was having shoulder pain. You don't realise, either, how much you miss an arm when you are eating and can't even cut things up. It is a very hard journey and not one to be made lightly. It's definitely not something you would put your body through if it wasn't needed.

The first look at my new piece was a few hours later when they came to check it had a pulse. My smile was immense. It was alive and looked massive, we both said. I made a joke about it having a tan because it was off my arm. I can't explain how it felt; I was ecstatic that the surgeon had done an amazing job. The nurse said there was a lot of swelling; my new penis had its own little bed; it was padded out, very well supported and needed to stay elevated. At this point I couldn't even feel my legs, let alone move anything apart from my arms.

The phallus had a catheter inside it, but not connected to anything. This was to keep open the new urethra and would be removed on the day I left hospital. I had a lot of sore areas, it wasn't just my arm, it was my buttocks. Both of them had been cut and stitched, as this is the skin that was taken to graft onto my arm. Of course, I now had a new piece between my legs, too, so everything was stitched and sore. They were amazing at managing pain, and kept me topped up all the time. I never had to ask for pain killers, they just brought them in for me at regular intervals. The phallus didn't look too stylish at that point. You could see my tattoo on the end, saying "my love", which both Julie and the nurse smiled at. This would not be seen eventually, as I would have glans sculpting, creating a 'head'. At present I was very happy. One of the best bits was when the nurse came in with a heartbeat monitor just like they use in maternity wards. She put it onto the phallus every half hour to hear the pulse, which was very strong. It is a great feeling, as then you know the surgery has worked, I just needed it to carry on for a few days to get out of the danger area. I was thrilled the surgery had worked, beaming from ear to ear, but everything was still numb. I managed to eat a sandwich later that night, and I started to get the feeling back in my legs at around 9pm – it's not nice when you can see your feet but can't even wiggle your toes. The nurses were amazing with my personal care and re-doing my dressings. I know it's a nurse's job, but these people always went above and beyond. They were so nice to talk to, and would stick their heads around the door just to see if I wanted anything. I didn't get a lot of sleep that night, with a lot of pain in my shoulder and the leg cuffs blowing up and down every ten minutes to keep circulation flowing. They brought me extra pain killers, urine was passing fine, drains were great, not losing too much, all was as good as could be. It seems I heal really well and quite quickly. The doctor called in and said everything was good, but they were keeping hourly checks on me as my blood pressure was still in the 80s and they wanted it higher. They advised me to drink more, and told me my blood group is A positive. I didn't have any feeling in my new piece, which concerned me at the time, but apparently this is to be expected and it can take up to twelve months to get any sensation. Each day I longed to hear that heartbeat which made me feel great inside and sure that all was working as it should be.

Day Two: there was a breakfast of bacon, eggs, the full works. Julie cut it up for me, and I wondered how I would manage when she went home! My observations were now carried out two hourly, which meant I got a bit more rest. The nurses came in and rolled me onto my side so they could check the stitches on my buttocks: very tidy, one nurse said. She had been right next to the surgeon in theatre and said it was really interesting to watch the procedure. They re-dressed my buttock wounds with some new strips, this time it felt sore when they were doing it – there is a risk of blistering when dressings are being changed. The old vaginal area also had to be cleaned, as part of this had been stitched in order to bury the clitoris. One nurse held my leg up whilst the other nurse cleaned and dressed the wounds.

The surgeon visited to say that the operation went well and he was pleased with the result. I would be staying in hospital for seven days and then sent home with medication and a letter for my GP. They would also contact my GP to arrange for district nurses to come to the house as getting to the surgery was not an option at first, when lower mobility would be very limited. Over the next couple of days, I developed a sore under my arm, from where it was resting against a pillow - ouch. The vaginal area was very swollen, too. When they say you will be bedridden for a couple of days, you can certainly understand why. We had decided that Julie should go home rather than sleep in the car, so one of our friends drove up with my daughter and picked Julie up; it was nice to see them both. We left my car in the car park so we would have transport home when she returned for me at the end of the week.

Antibiotics were given intravenously, but this was very uncomfortable, and I found that the quicker it went in the more painful it was. The nurse said that if the liquid went in too fast it would cause discomfort. They took the cannula out of my hand and I took my medication orally. I had a bed bath on day two, which was slightly awkward, and they changed the bed sheets. I still felt sore in a lot of places.

Day Three: this was the first morning without Julie. I had slept better, my observation checks moved from two hourly to four hourly, though they kept the light on all night! My blood pressure was still low. Breakfast arrived and I was looking forward to it. The first thing I realised was my left arm was up in the air and I couldn't use it, Julie had helped with everything until then, but now I had to do it myself and I was struggling. I couldn't cut anything, and even when taking out a tea bag or opening a sugar sachet I realised how hard things are without two arms. I had the daily injection into my stomach which I had been having since the operation, to stop blood clotting. It is only a tiny needle but stings for about sixty seconds when they administer it. I was told I would have to administer it myself for twenty-one days after I was discharged. It sounds silly when my body has been through such amazing journeys, but I am scared of a little bloody needle and the thought of doing it to myself made me sweat. Maybe Julie would do this for me?

A nurse came to check my observations and give me a bed bath. I can't remember how the conversation started but she didn't realise what I was in for; she thought I was born male and was in hospital for a penis extension, as she cares for a lot of men that have that done. She praised me and commented that she would never have known, and that I had blown her away. She said I had more muscle and looked better than a real man - I wasn't too sure about the "Real Man" bit, but didn't take offence, although I know some people would. She was there to care and look after me, and kept saying I had shocked her and it was a miracle. She was in my room for over forty five minutes. I am not sure she should have been there that long but she was intrigued and asked so many questions. She said it was the first time she had cared for a transman and she was honoured, asking my previous name and my current name, reassuring me that she wouldn't touch any of my wounds. It's natural for people to be interested.

The surgeon, Dr. G, came to see me and said that once I got up and walked around, so they could check I wouldn't lose any blood, I could possibly have my drain out. This pleased me, as I felt I had several little handbags to carry around. Dr. G. is a man of few words but is a great surgeon, answered anything I asked, and was really pleased with my progress. He wanted me to get up and walk to the shower that afternoon. My first thought was, "You've got no chance of me getting out of this bed just yet." I couldn't even sit up without help. However, if that's what I was asked to do I was determined to do it. I am not one to sit and mope, but didn't think it would happen.

It was around 11am when I really needed to open my bowels. As I couldn't get up yet, I would have to ask for a bed pan. I had been having lactulose to make it easier. I had a buzzer but felt silly and didn't want to ask. I knew the nurses dealt with this every day, but I didn't like the idea of a bed pan. However, trying to hold it was making me really hot and sick, and giving me belly ache, so I had to call. In came the cardboard bed pan. Could I go? Could I buggery! The pan was hard and a strange shape, which lifted the area - so uncomfortable on my stitches. It was not happening, and I found myself tensing. I just didn't want to go whilst lying in bed. That useless feeling returned, and I found myself getting upset. After a while, the feeling of wanting to go went away. I wanted a drink but knew it would make me want to go again and figured that pretty soon I would be getting up for my shower.

At about 1pm the nurses came to give me a bed bath. I was feeling tired, the leg cuffs, called Veniflow, kept my circulation flowing and were continually blowing up and down. The nurses chatted with me as if they were my long lost friends, and remarked on the amazing surgery, which gave me so much confidence. If I had been asked to score my pain from 1-10, I would have said 1: I felt really good. I was a bit worried that I wouldn't understand everything the nurses told me, or wouldn't remember it. I mentioned this, and the nurses said I could always ring up the ward and ask them over the phone, which was reassuring. I recorded most conversations on my phone as I know my memory is terrible and wanted to re-listen to what was said to me. The nurses all said they loved their job and the place they worked. One of the nurses looked at my drains and said I had only drained 140ml which was brilliant. That day was the anniversary of my chest surgery and one nurse commented that my chest and the tattoo covering my scar lines looked great. I bet they were washing and drying me and changing my dressings for about an hour. When it came to changing my buttock dressings I needed the side of the bed to be up so I could hold onto it for a bit of support. After cleaning me, the nurses changed all the bedding, ordered me a cup of tea, and I slept for an hour.

At around 5.30pm, when the next nursing shift began, the nurses came in and lowered the bed. They helped me get my legs out, complete with sexy stockings. On the count of three they helped me to stand; my blood pressure was really low, still in the 80s when they wanted it over 100; they told me to keep breathing as, with low blood pressure, you can pass out after being in bed for a few days. I felt slightly light headed and sweaty handed but I was told this was to be expected. The first stop was the commode but I struggled to lower myself as I couldn't use my left arm. I sat down eventually, but still couldn't go to the toilet. I think I needed privacy, to be honest. After five minutes they walked me to the toilet.

I stood and started to walk. Very tiny steps, but I was doing it, on my own as well. There were tubes everywhere, down below, so I had to be careful. I had a catheter in the end of my phallus, plus a drain at either side of my groin and another catheter collecting my urine. The nurses helped me to sit on the toilet then left me there for a while; it was a strange feeling as tubes were everywhere. I wanted to go, and started pushing, but stopped, as it felt as if everything was going to fall out. After sitting there for quite a while, I opened my bowels without pushing - what a relief that was! Now I was looking forward to that lovely shower with the water running all over me. I called the nurses to tell them I had been, and they came in to get me, but explained I had to go back to the chair and wouldn't be having a shower that day because my drains had not been taken out. I was very disappointed as I so wanted a shower, a daily wipe down is not what I like, but I couldn't do much about it. They took me back to a chair where I sat there doing some colouring and watching television for a couple of hours, but sitting upright started to make my buttock stitches hurt, so when they came to give me my medication, they moved me back to bed so the pressure was off my buttocks.

My dinner was brought in - steak and chips followed by ice cream. I looked at it and wondered how on earth I was going to be able to cut up the steak. I stabbed it and tried to eat. The ice cream was in a tub. I managed to get the lid off with my teeth, only to find there was a plastic film over the top of it. I pulled with my teeth and it ripped, I pulled around the other side and it ripped again. Three times I tried to get the bloody lid off, it was just not happening, so no ice cream. When they collected my tray I pointed out, nicely, that I hadn't been able to open it, and within five minutes a tub of ice cream, minus the lid, appeared on my table; the staff were very helpful and obliging.

I had spoken to Julie several times during the day. I felt good in myself, but tired, so even if she had been there I probably wouldn't have been great company. I nodded off quite early that night.

Day 4: I slept well through the night, apart from continuing four hourly observations as my blood pressure did not seem to be getting any higher. The nurses advised me to drink more water to bring it up, but also thought it had a lot to do with lying in bed doing nothing and not moving. They also gave me my medication through the night, to keep me comfortable – so I was sore, but not in pain.

When the nurses changed my buttock dressings, they noticed that the dressing around the vagina had quite a bit of blood on it. This was the first time anyone had actually looked in that region, they had checked the new penis and his heartbeat, but hadn't looked underneath, where the vagina still was. The nurse commented that I had a few blisters down there as well; it wasn't bleeding, so must have been blood from surgery. I had been prepared 'down there' for my next stage, and had a hole where the urethra would be joined up next time. The nurse told me that I would be taught how to inject my stomach, that day, which stopped me in my tracks. I was most definitely not looking forward to that, and didn't want to learn. I explained that I would like Julie to learn to do the injections and she wouldn't be back until the next day. The nurse said this would be okay, and they would show Julie when she came. After all I had been through, I couldn't bring myself to put a little needle in me.

A male nurse came to take out my catheter and one of my drains, so I could have my shower. Oh yes, it's shower time, I thought, but first the catheter and drain had to come out, which was going to hurt. I asked one of the nurses to video it for me so I could look back on things. The male nurse taking out the bits was lovely, but I struggled to understand some of the things he was saying, so I would look at the female nurse and she would explain. My bum stitches were feeling very sore that day, and the nurse explained that as I was now sitting up more, and as they went all around both thighs, there was more pressure being applied in that area. He walked towards me with a syringe, without a needle in it, and I asked what it was for. He explained that there was something that resembles a small balloon filled with saline keeping the catheter in place inside, and that he was going to drain out the saline with the syringe, allowing the catheter to slide out. This sounded easy and painless. He put the end of the syringe into the tube and sucked out the saline; there was a strange sensation, as though I was going to wet myself. He showed me the end of it. Wow, I thought, one less tube in me.

    Next was the drain. I still had two of these, one each side of me. He went over to his table and brought over a little packet. As he opened it my eyebrows rose. "What is that," I asked? "It's a Stanley blade," he replied. It's funny how you can feel sick and very hot just by looking at something. I laughed, I knew he wasn't there to hurt me. He started to peel off the very sticky plaster that was stuck to my very hairy legs. The female nurse, videoing, was laughing and saying it was like being waxed. He got his little blade and seemed to take forever to cut through the stitches to pull out the drain. I felt very nervous, hot and anxious, and asked them both to keep talking to me, to take my mind off what he was doing. He told me to take a deep breath and I felt myself tense up as he pulled out the drain. There was a tugging feeling, but it was out. He asked me if I want to see it, which I did. The part that had been inside me was about six inches long.

He applied a pad to stop any bleeding and I put my thumb up to the camera to ask the nurse to stop filming. I felt a bit queasy.

It was now time to head for that shower I had been waiting for. They put a big plastic sleeve over my arm to stop the dressings getting wet, and I walked to the bathroom. A towel was placed next to the shower tray to stop me from slipping, and I stepped into the shower. I still had one 'handbag' left, which was the drain leading to a big plastic bottle, so that was placed on the shower tray floor as I got in. I stood there with two nurses; the water was turned on and it was running down my head and back. I stood there with my eyes closed, relishing this lovely feeling of getting clean. one nurse poured shower gel onto my hand and I washed my hair and face. I could wash the top of my body one side, but as I couldn't use my left arm I needed some help. There were traces of blood in the tray, from down below, and the nurses gave me a cleansing wipe to wash myself downstairs. I mentioned it felt sore and lumpy around my stitches and they assured me that was normal. My shower came to an end and they dried me. I could do some bits, but it is so hard without the use of one arm. The nurse peeled off a couple of dressings whilst they were wet.

I was taken back to my bed, where all my dressings and gauze were re-done, apart from my arm. My new penis was cleaned underneath and around the base where it is stitched into place. I didn't have any feeling in it, but the nurse explained that it would take time for the nerves to heal. The area looked very tidy without dressings. The base of the phallus was damp, and the nurse dabbed it with gauze, using tweezers, saying he needed to keep an eye on that area, as sometimes you can develop something called a fistula where the skin breaks away at the base. I didn't like the sound of that, but he said it all looked good to him. I noticed he put more gauze at the base, to soak up moisture. It is quite a difficult dressing, as it has to go completely around the base. The phallus was put back on several pads, so it stayed at an angle of 45 degrees, as they don't want it hanging down. They also have to put a dressing on the underside of the phallus, as that was completely stitched too. I still had a catheter in the end of the penis to keep the urethra open. The nurse brought out the heart beat monitor and that put a smile on my face. He confirmed that the veins, arteries and oxygen supply were all working and healing well.

The rest of the day went quite quickly. I did some colouring and watched the television. I felt I had a bit more freedom now I wasn't stuck in bed. However, when I dropped my pen and book onto the floor I couldn't get down to pick them up and just sat there and waited for twenty minutes as I was not going to call the nurses in for that! Eventually, a nurse brought in a sharps box for me to put used needles in at home, so she kindly picked up my book and pen and helped me back to the bed, as I was getting tired. I drifted in and out of sleep, ate my dinner and saw some lovely nurses and canteen staff, who popped their heads round the door to say hello. I had my medication, and my observations were now six hourly so I was looking forward to a real good night's sleep.

Later on, when I went for a wee, it felt strange. I was sitting on the toilet with both bits, and weeing from the old bits. I also found that I wet my dressings when I weed, as it ran down my thigh, so the poor nurses had to re-dress my buttock dressings each time, which was a bit embarrassing. I tried opening my legs wider, but it didn't work. Not only that, the urine was stinging my skin graft, which was getting me down. I went to sleep early and I was looking forward to tomorrow already, as Julie was coming to see me. I had missed her so much.

Day 5: I woke up at 6.30am for my medication and morning stomach injection, feeling on top of the world. It had been strange being apart from Julie, but I had been tired and slept a lot, so I think I needed the rest. My breakfast was brought in at 8.30am, but I wasn't feeling too well by then. I felt sick and woozy, so I had two mouthfuls of breakfast so I could take more medication, and only drank half a cup of tea, which is unlike me. I had been okay until I had the first lot of meds. Hoping I would feel better later, I went back to sleep for a while. At lunchtime, two nurses come back in to take out my final drain. That Stanley blade came towards me again, and the nurse said she was going to cut the stitches close to the skin, so she had more to pull it out towards her. Unlike the day before, this happened quite quickly, so I didn't have time to think about it. Afterwards, she applied pressure to the area, then moved onto my phallus. I wasn't sure what she was doing, but she was cutting the stitches around the catheter. I was surprised, as I had thought this would be left in, but she assured me it had to go. She cut the stitches and gently pulled on the tube. It seemed to be sticking slightly, but she kept on coaxing and pulling and eventually it started to move. It was a long piece of tubing and when it was out I was tube free and feeling better by the minute. She lifted up my phallus and said my stitches were very red, and asked if the surgeon had seen them, but I hadn't seen him since my shower.

The day went really slowly. I wasn't expecting Julie until around 5pm. but felt a lot better when I knew she had left home. I had some lovely lunch and sat in my chair, but didn't have a shower, as it isn't good to keep getting the dressings wet. Julie arrived around 4.30pm and my face lit up, I had missed her so much. Our friend had brought her back and she was going to stay in the car that night, then we would be driving back in our own car when I was discharged the next day. I think she was really happy to see how much I had come on in a few days, she came over and hugged and kissed me. I rang through to the canteen and ordered some tea and sandwiches. As I have said before, this was more like a hotel than a hospital. Julie and I spent the afternoon chatting and catching up, even though we had spoken daily on the phone. More medication arrived, which kept me virtually pain free. Eventually our friend left for home. The nurse who I spoke to regarding injections to my stomach came to say hello, and explained that she would come back in the morning, to show Julie how to do it. That made me nervous; we joked that if I got on Julie's nerves she would jab me, but I knew she wouldn't hurt me on purpose. Eventually Julie went back to the car, we chatted by phone, then both went to sleep.

101

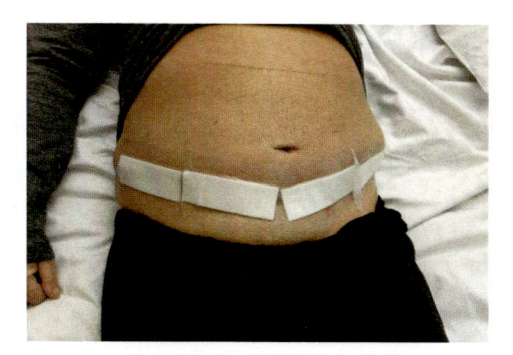

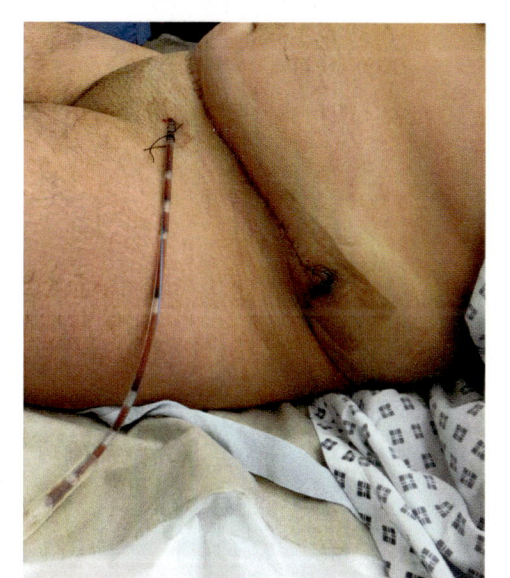

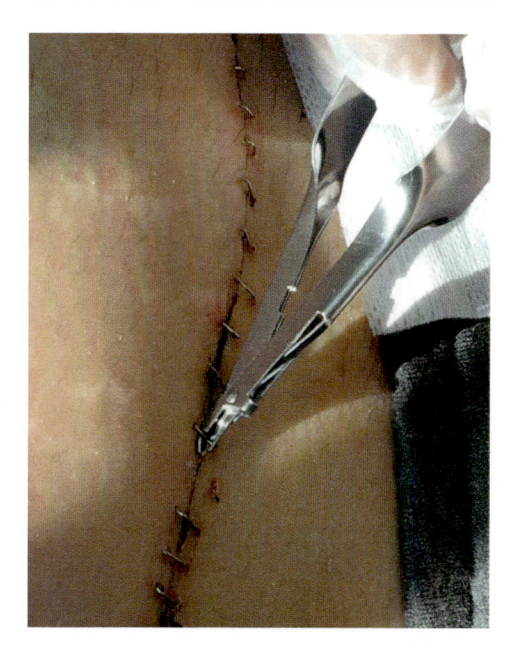

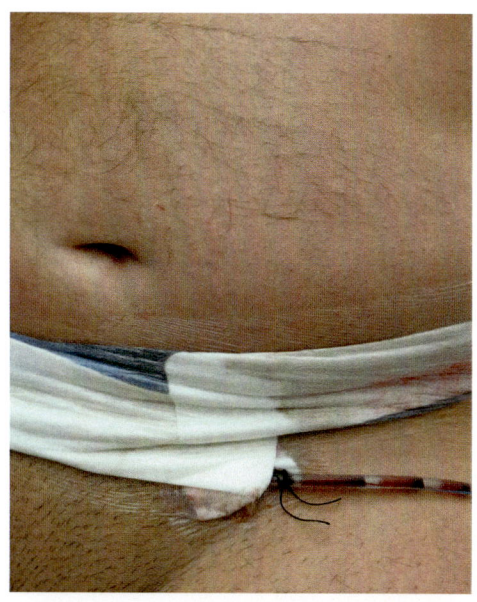

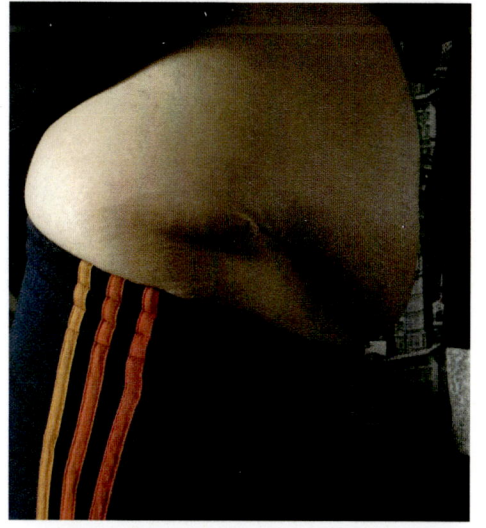

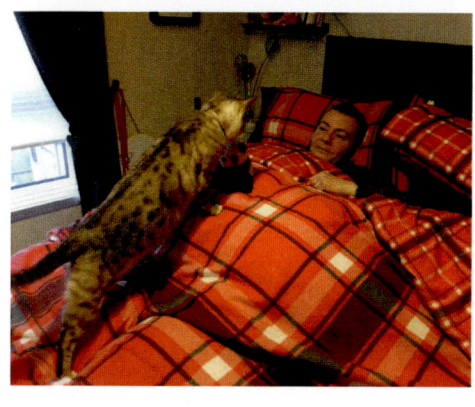

103

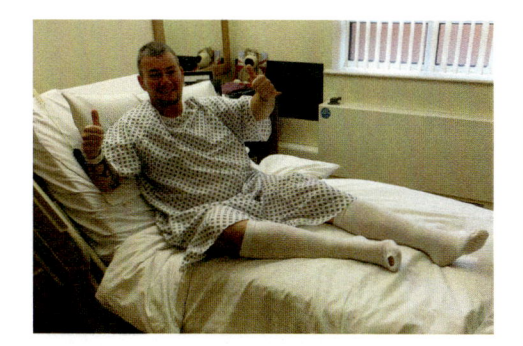

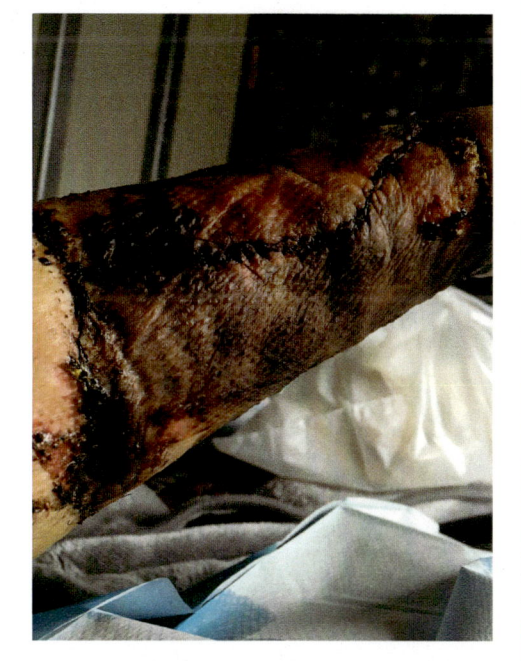

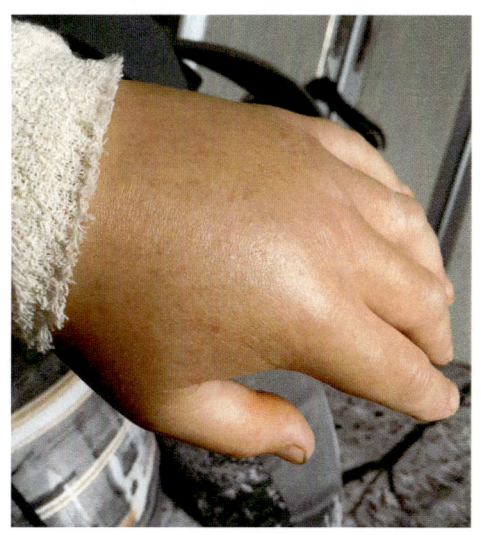

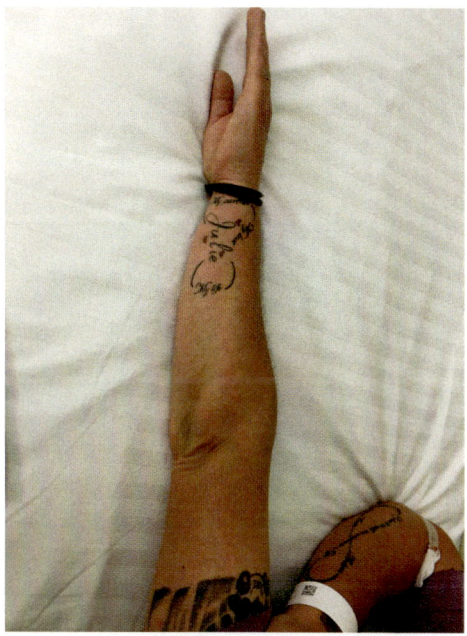

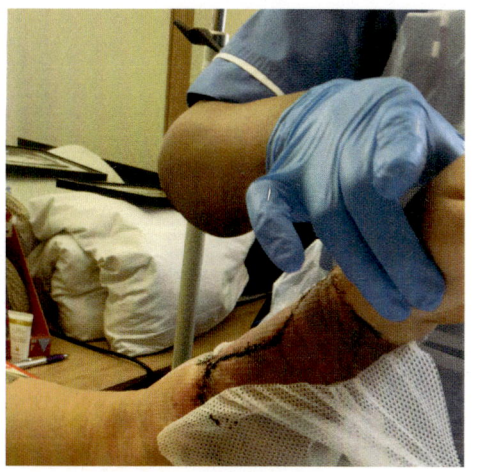

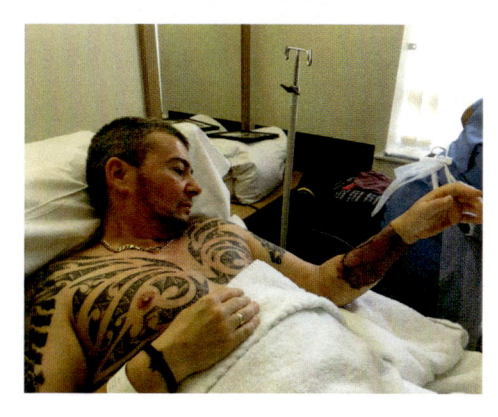

Chapter Fifteen

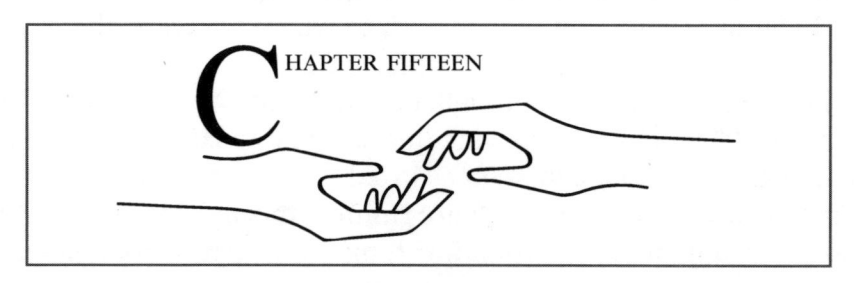

Discharged

Day 6: It was discharge day, 6.30am, and medication arrived. Julie came in around 7.00am having been in the car all night. Breakfast was at 8.00am, for Julie, too. The nurse came in to teach Julie how to give me my injection. Here we go, I thought, but Julie was told what to do and just did it, and to be honest it didn't feel any different to a nurse doing it. Phew!

The bandages were coming off my left arm, that day, for them to have a look. This was going to be the first time I would see it; I didn't know what I was expecting or how I would feel. Bit by bit, the bandage was unravelled. A couple of layers in and I could see the blood where it had seeped through. In certain areas this made removing the bandage hard work. I asked if I was going to see the area which had been operated on. "Yes," said the nurse, it was all coming off. Did I want to see it? Some people don't. I knew it wasn't going to be very pleasant, but I was intrigued and wanted to see my arm. At one point the dressing was sticking so much that she pulled my arm. She wasn't rough, but it was enough to make me jerk, and that hurt. She started to use some scissors, as the bandage just wasn't unravelling anymore. There was quite a lot of bruising on my bicep and underneath my arm, I was also struggling to move my second and third finger, and when I did, there was a sharp shooting pain straight through the back of my hand. I was starting to feel very sick and hot. She still wasn't having too much luck, so they decided to put me in the shower.

As the dressing got wet it would be easier to remove. She joked that it could take us all day to get my dressings off.

I had my shower and I was back to where we were about an hour before, only this time the bandage was coming off easily. The final piece of bandage unravelled, and I said, "Wow, that looks very neat." I had someone videoing this and looking back at the video, the minute I said "Wow," I told them to stop the camera. I'm not sure what emotions were running through me, obviously no one wants to see a wound, I think I was just overwhelmed. There was a lot of swelling to my hand; it looked huge, wax like, and very shiny. I couldn't make a fist and could only move my fingers very slightly. If I tried to clench it, a painful spasm shot down the back of my hand, and when they pressed on the back of it we could see fluid under the skin. I had done this to myself for a very good reason - to make me happy and complete. The surgeon had already said everything had gone well, so I'm not sure what I should have been expecting, but I was happy. I knew it would take time, but that a good tattoo would eventually cover this. Julie thought it looked sore, which it did, but it was tidy and clean. I already knew that I healed well, so hopefully it would be the same this time round.

They cleaned all around my arm and started to re-dress it. The first thing that was applied was something called Jelonet, a gel coating that heals wounds. They wrapped this all around the new skin graft. I found it quite hard and tiring to hold my arm whilst it was being dressed. I was aching and the more I moved it the more I hurt. After the Jelonet, the nurse applied square pieces of normal gauze dressing, then a bandage was applied over the top of those. I couldn't take my eyes off what they were doing and how my arm was looking; I don't think I had been prepared for how my arm would look, but I was okay. I tried to straighten my arm but it just was not happening. It hurt to move it, but they told me in time it would straighten. After all, I had had major surgery only a few days ago. After the very neat dressing, the nurse applied tape to hold it into place. Then she moved onto the buttocks;

cleaning the wounds and applying new dressings over the stitches – this had already happened several times, as every time I weed, the dressings got wet. Then for the phallus. As she lifted it up to have a look underneath, she noticed there was blood trickling down. Panic crept in, and they didn't know why there was a steady trickle. The person recording this was asked to stop filming. I commented that something between my legs was stinging. I was getting concerned. Why was I bleeding? The nurse pressed on one side of my pubic bone area and said one side was very hard and the other side wasn't, but this was in the groin, not underneath my new piece. It was with reference to that area that a previous nurse had mentioned the word fistula. The area was very dark, as blood had collected there. That part of the skin had not taken, so blood has to find its way out of somewhere. It pushed itself out of the stitches, and was now making its way out of me. I knew the part of my skin where it was attached had not taken, and had died, or was dying. I felt so upset, and worried everything I had just gone through would be wasted, but the good thing was I had a pulse in my phallus, so that was still alive. A fistula is apparently very common and nothing to worry about, as another skin graft during the next operation can fix it. Sometimes a bit of tissue can be taken from inside the mouth or somewhere else and be grafted on, so it's not the end of the world, but I didn't know that as I lay on my hospital bed. They padded out my groin and dressed my wounds; these would be checked again before I went home. I was looking forward to being back in my own environment. Julie packed my stuff whilst we enjoyed chatting to each other, and the rest of the morning went really fast. I felt good in myself and apart from the bleeding, everything was great and I was healing well. During my stay at the hospital, I had felt very comfortable, at ease and well looked after; I couldn't have been anywhere nicer. I was over the moon with how the surgery went and the very good results.

 The nurse brought my discharge letter and medication and explained what would happen next. She gave me a leaflet about

DVT (Deep Vein Thrombosis) and said I would have to wear the sexy stockings for the next seven days. The discharge letter listed my medication and the nurse explained the pink copy had to be dropped into the GP, though she would personally be calling my surgery to explain the medication and what dressings I would be needing. She gave me a box of clexane 40mg, which was my daily injection into the stomach. There were eight left in the box. Codeine phosphate and paracetamol could be taken when needed, co-amoxiclav antibiotic had to be taken three times per day for nine days, and a bottle of lactulose 15ml (which I called my Baileys) three times per day. I was told not to knock my arm or rotate it in any way for about three weeks. A district nurse would visit every day to change my dressings down below, and once a week to change the one on my arm. The nurse also told me I had an appointment booked for 15th July, at 145 Harley Street, and I would receive confirmation of this in the post. That was it; I was free to go!

They brought a wheelchair to my room and I was wheeled to reception, where I thanked all the staff on duty for looking after me so well. I managed to get out of my chair and took a few steps outside, to where Julie had brought the car. Getting in and lowering myself down was difficult, but once seated I was okay for a while. Sitting upright made my buttocks sore, where they were stitched, but as we set off on the hour and a half journey home I was looking forward to seeing our animals and to being able to sleep in a bed next to my missus.

We made it home without me moaning too much about my backside. I felt I had no energy at all, but I had been in bed for quite a few days. Julie made a protective 'cage' to put around me, like she did after the first op. I sat in the lounge for a while but started to feel uncomfortable and wanted to lie down to take the pressure off my buttocks. I found the stairs challenging; once I was up there I didn't want to come back downstairs. The first night was quite awkward as I sleep on the right side of the bed which meant my left arm was right next to Julie. I was frightened of knocking it, but didn't want to sleep on the left in case the cats jumped up and caught it. My arm had to be up in the air so we had cushions and pillows propping me up. I had an extra-long catheter tube, so the one that was on my thigh was plugged into another one that sat on the floor. I had to remember to empty it. It had a flip flow valve, so when the bag was full I could pull the lever and it emptied.

The following morning I felt sick, but I think that was because of having my meds without eating. Julie had a look at my dressings and I was still bleeding down below. Julie re-dressed the area and explained there was bleeding from a hole the size of a five pence coin cut in half. She told me to ring the doctor first thing, which I did. I informed the receptionist I had just come out of hospital and my dressings had fallen off; she went off somewhere, then came back, saying that according to my notes I was mobile, so I had to get in myself to the surgery. I knew this was virtually impossible, as I struggled to get up the stairs, let alone to the surgery. I explained I couldn't really walk, and the district nurse rang me back. After we spoke, she said she would come out to me, so I just had to wait until she arrived. She couldn't give me a time but she would be there at some point. Julie left a packed lunch, a flask of tea, the tv remote and a colouring book by my bed, and said she would be back later. I slept on and off and got myself to the bathroom to have a wash and clean my teeth. It was hard and uncomfortable to sit on the toilet. I tried to get in the shower, but couldn't, as it is in our bath and I couldn't get my leg that high by myself. Julie had already said she would shower me when she got back, but it was frustrating. I'm not used to being in bed and found lying around quite stressful. I wanted to do things, but my body wasn't letting me. I was never one to ask for help, but right now I was relying on Julie for everything.

The nurse arrived at around 2.30pm. She went through the notes, then removed the dressings from around my phallus. "Boy, that's big," she said. I had to laugh. She hadn't done any dressings like this before, "but a wound is a wound," she said. We had a chat, which made me feel at ease. In hospital I had felt okay because I know the nurses deal with these dressings on a daily basis, whereas district nurses don't come across this sort of thing that often. The nurse was pleasant, though. She couldn't understand why on earth I had been declared mobile, and said she would be visiting me for some time yet. She wrote in my folder and said she would be back on the Wednesday, and would change my arm dressing too, so I would get to see that after a week. Within an hour of the nurse leaving, my dressing had fallen off, and I hadn't even got out of bed.

Julie came home and helped me into the shower. She had bought a long plastic sleeve to go over my arm, because that couldn't get wet. I got into the shower and that was nice, but getting out was a different matter. I couldn't reach to put my foot down onto the floor and this upset me, I couldn't sit on the edge of the bath either, because my stitches hurt. We ended up putting a small step the other side of the bath and I leaned on Julie to kind of pull myself out so she could dry and dress me. I was feeling pretty useless, and cried a lot when I was alone.

The following morning the district nurse rang me to check on yesterday's dressings. When I told her they had fallen off and Julie had to redo them, she said she would come out again that day. She also asked if I minded a student nurse coming with her, to learn, as it's not every day you get a patient like me. I said it wouldn't bother me at all as long as I was being cared for. They arrived and again we chatted. The nurse re-dressed me down below, then decided she was ready to look at my arm. She didn't know what she was expecting and neither did I. As she started to unravel the dressings, I wanted to take pictures. When the dressing was off I was pleased; it looked better than last time I had seen it. It was, however, slightly scabby, whereas before it hadn't been. It reminded me of snake skin. The nurse assured me this was a sign of healing. She said I had put myself through the mill, but I didn't see this as it was what I had wanted. The hospital had told me a bit of gauze must be wrapped around my arm prior to a dressing going on, and had sent me home with some alginate. Once the nurse had used it she wrote it down and ordered some for the following week. I still couldn't clench my fist. When the dressings around my phallus were removed the base was quite wet, and the nurse reiterated what the hospital had said about a fistula. That really worried and upset me, as in my head, all I heard was skin dying and I thought things were going to die and not heal. I took pictures and emailed them over to St. Peter's Andrology. They responded with "All looks good", and said that if a fistula did appear there would be nothing to worry about as this could be fixed at my next surgery. That reassured me. My vaginal area was still really sore as well, and that tended to get missed. I had a new bit that needed looking after, but the old part was all stitched up and needed care. My hand was still very swollen and didn't seem to be going down at all. When I mentioned this to the hospital, they told me a compression glove would do the trick if I could get my GP to issue one. I contacted my surgery but they couldn't find one, so I bought one online, but it didn't seem to work. The nurse told me to give it time; she was pleased with my arm. She applied some of the alginate dressing and said she would do it again the following week.

During that afternoon my arm felt really tight and my hand was throbbing. It felt as if the nurse had put the bandage on too tight. By the time Julie got home my hand was even bigger and all the little veins in it had broken. Julie undid the bandage as far as the alginate dressing and re-dressed my arm. I felt instant relief, but unfortunately the veins had already broken and the hand didn't look very nice.

I was upset, as none of this had arisen from the actual surgery, but by a dressing being applied too tightly. At the time I thought it would settle down, but eighteen months later I still have the broken veins in my hand. One of the hardest things during transition is that once we have had an operation we are treated and cared for by a GP or local district nurse who isn't fully aware of what we have gone through.

CHAPTER SIXTEEN

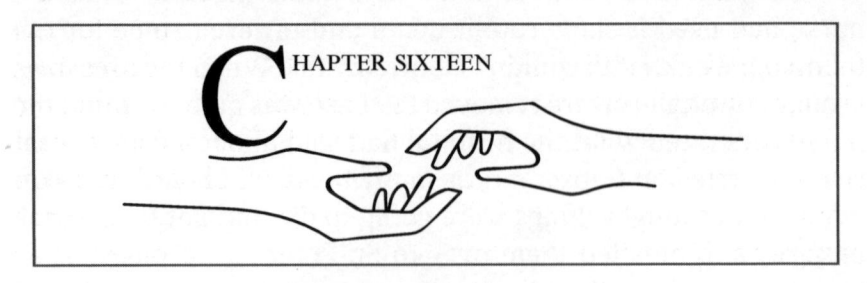

Two Weeks Later

By this time, I was moving a lot more easily. I still had no feeling in the phallus and on its underside there was still a hole, which seemed to be getting bigger. Julie was dressing this every day and the nurse was coming out every other day. My arm wasn't a pretty sight; it was very red and looked as if I had been badly burned, but the nurse said it was healing well. My buttocks, across the creases, and inner and outer thigh, were also healing, though sitting was still really sore. The nurse ordered me a memory foam cushion, helping me to sit more comfortably without slouching to avoid putting pressure directly on the stitches. Instead of the big dressings on my buttocks, which needed changing often because I was still wetting them when going to the toilet, she gave me a spray waterproof plaster. This was amazing, as now I wasn't getting so wet and sore because it didn't absorb, so Julie could wash me in the morning, spray this on and it would last throughout the day, brilliant! The phallus was looking good on three sides, but the hole was causing concern. It was purple, and the nurse told me the skin had died in that area. Although the possibility had been mentioned before, to be told it has actually happened is quite shocking. I rang the hospital and explained what I had been told, and they asked me to email over some pictures. They got back to me within twenty minutes. The pictures had been shown to a surgeon, who replied that all looked healthy, and that it looked as if I had lost several stitches, causing the hole to be as big as it was. He said it was nothing to worry about as this would be corrected at my next surgery. My Harley Street review had been arranged for 22nd July, but they didn't want to wait until then, so they made me an appointment for 5th July – the following week. I contacted my GP and asked if he could prescribe me some painkillers, as on discharge they only gave me a week's supply. I wasn't in lots of pain, but I wanted something to take the edge off at times as my arm still ached. I could now do the stairs a lot more easily and comfortably, one step at a time.

5th July

I arrived at Harley Street. It was the first time I had ever been on this road and, from what I knew, it was a very rich place where only wealthy people went. We went through big front doors, into a very big building. At the reception area I was told to go downstairs and that someone would be with me shortly. It was a small waiting area and there were two other transmen waiting to be seen. When it was my time to be called in to see the nurse, she talked to me and read my notes, then showed me to the couch. I took down my trousers for her to examine the area and she confirmed I did have a fistula, that part of my skin had died and had not attached as it should, but said that it was nothing at all to worry about as this is completely fixable. She said the area looked clean and there was no discharge. There was a blister at the top of the phallus, but this was reducing and looked dry. With regards to the arm graft, the blisters covering this area had now been fully adsorbed. There was a small site near the crease of my elbow that looked slightly wet, which was cleaned with saline and redressed with kaltostat on the wet area and mepitel on the rest of the healthy tissue and then covered with gauze and crepe bandage. The nurse reported that my buttock area was healing really well and was clean and dry. This was all a relief. I was pleased I went, just for peace of mind. She re-dressed the areas, then had a look at my arm to see how that was healing, and said she was impressed. The plan was for a further appointment in two weeks, to flush out the neourethra and pass a LoFric catheter. I wasn't there very long, but long enough to know I was doing fine. Julie drove us back home.

I went to work with Julie a few times that next week, just to get out of the house and to see people. My kids had been round, all four of them, but I hadn't seen my dad, so we saw him, and my aunty came to visit us at the garage. I was still struggling with my hand; even after four weeks, and if I moved my fingers I got a shooting pain. I guessed it could be nerve damage. My hand was still very swollen and looked like a fake hand – waxy.

22nd July 2016 – 5 weeks post op

I was back for another visit at Harley Street, and for my dressings to be changed again. I was now walking and moving a lot better. The dissolvable stitches in my buttocks were nearly all gone, but my phallus was monitored more closely. The nurse inspected the areas: the arm had healed well, with just a small moist area requiring alginate dressing; the phallus had healed, although a urethrocutaneous fistula was evident at the base, which would be addressed at my next surgery; the buttock wounds had healed well, with no areas of breakdown. The nurse had a plastic tube (16 french catheter) that she pushed into the end of the penis and fed down via the neo-urethra. You could see it pass by the area where the skin hadn't formed correctly and the edge of the plastic tube came out of a little hole they had created for my next stage, where they would join up the urethra. This was done to make sure the new urethra hadn't closed up. There were no problems, all was looking good and she was very happy with how I was healing. She provided me with a 20ml syringe in order to flush the neo-urethra until my next surgery, she also told me I was ready to go on the waiting list for my next stage – exciting!

24th July

I could have my first soak in the bath, wow, this was lush! I could just lie there. Julie asked me what I thought as I looked down at myself. Obviously very different from when I last had a bath, I said. To me, my phallus just looked like an add-on at the moment, not real, more like a huge, plain sausage. There was no head and no sculpting yet, so it didn't look very natural and you could see all the stitches where it had been positioned. On a positive note, placed where it was, I couldn't see any of the female parts which were still there and didn't seem normal at all.

My bath was full of salt to try and heal all my wounds. They recommend bathing for around twenty minutes at a time, I didn't realise this and was in for over an hour, but nothing bad happened. As I was lying in the bath, I could see my arm scabs starting to lift off, not a pretty site but it did look so much better without scabs. I still had a few stitches there, which were dissolving over time, but my arm still felt really tight. My hand was still swollen and when you pressed the back of it, you could tell there was still fluid there as it took a long time for the skin to rise. The nurse had instructed me to take an open-ended syringe (without a needle) put it into the bath and draw some salted bath water up into it. I had to put the tip of the syringe into the tip of the penis and gently press the syringe downwards. The water would be expelled into the penis and would run out of the little hole that was created for the new urethra hook up. This was to make sure the inside of the new phallus was kept clean, as at present there was nothing in it. When I first started doing this, the water coming out was rather cloudy due to bits of blood being present, but after doing it in the bath for a few days, the water cleared. This was to be continued daily until stage 2. I was feeling so good lying in the bath, I didn't want to get out. Julie helped me out and dried me down, then re-dressed everywhere. I am so lucky to have her. The nurse had told me a salt bath every day would help, so I was already looking forward to tomorrow night. My bottom was still sore, especially when I sat on a hard chair. Once I got out the bath I was feeling really good and tried on my boxers without any dressings on. Just posing, to see what I looked like. I felt great.

That day, we had gone on a car journey, and it was the first time I had been able to drive using both hands, so that made my day. I was on the move. After an hour in the car though, I would get a bit fidgety, and I was still struggling with the rotation of my arm, which felt like it didn't want to turn and had very restricted movement. My hand was still very swollen, too.

28th July 2016

The district nurse came out to see me again. She now came on a weekly basis, to change the dressing on my arm and find out what other dressings we needed for the week. It had been decided that Julie would change my dressings down below, as she was re-doing them every other day anyway. I hadn't seen the nurse since I started to have salt baths, so she would see how I was healing. I was really impressed with how the bath helped, because I saw it daily now, whereas the nurse didn't. The scabs were coming off naturally; I was just letting my arm soak. If the scabs seemed loose I would gently wash that area and they would flake off. We were on week four following the operation and I was back to my normal routine, going to work daily, not lifting any heavy stuff, and being careful not to bang my arm, which was in a sling as it had to be kept raised. My hand was still very swollen, however, and showed no signs of reducing.

Daily life carried on and each day I felt better and better, but I was still getting a lot of pain in the back of my swollen hand when I clenched my fist or wiggled my fingers. One of the hardest things you deal with emotionally, is what you assume others will think and say behind your back, and this did play a massive part. Once back at work I was asked what I had done to my arm, as it was bandaged up and in a sling. I just said I had had a skin graft, which was the truth. It does make you feel uncomfortable - not because you don't believe in what you're doing but because you don't know what response you will get, and it puts you on edge. I have heard this from others, too. I have to say, though, that not one person has ever said anything bad to me. One person asked me what I had done, then asked what sort of skin graft, and why? Initially, I froze, then I just told him. He said, "Wow, really? That's amazing!" and asked a lot more questions. Before he left, he asked for some business cards and said he would promote my company at his work place. Since then, although I will not come out with it, if someone asks me a question I will not hide behind a lie or bend the truth. People have only ever been intrigued and said how brave I am for doing this and putting my body through it. It is something very serious, not just a fashion exchange because you want something different. It is real and can be life threatening. I don't have people asking anymore, as I am complete, look male and get called mate, geezer, buddy or fella. It feels great, but during the initial transition period it is awkward. My advice? Just hold your head high and don't let thoughts worry you.

10th August 2016
I had an appointment with a senior consultant back at Harley street, to see how I was doing, and if I could be put onto the waiting list for my next stage. The nurse had already said she was quite happy with moving me forward, but this needed to be approved by a surgeon. I had not seen this consultant before - a lovely chap. He examined me and was impressed with how I was healing. He commented that I still had a lot of swelling on my hand and recommended a compression glove, saying he would write to my GP. He measured my hand for the glove, which, to be honest, I had already bought. He also commented on the breakdown at the bottom of the phallus. He mentioned that my girth was quite big, and asked if Julie and I were happy with this. If not, I could have another operation to have this reduced if I wanted, but I really didn't want more operations than I needed to have. I wasn't having any problems and I didn't want to cause any either. We both liked what I had, so both said we were quite happy with the results. The consultant mentioned that, at my final stage, they planned to incorporate two cylinders along with my erectile device. He was happy for me to move forward to my next stage,

and I would be ready for this from 1st September onwards. The minimum break between any surgery is three months, allowing healing time, but as the waiting list is long, there could be almost a year between operations, unless I wanted to go on a cancellation list. As I have the flexibility, due to having my own company, I jumped at the chance of this. September was only a month away, and I had only just got back on my feet, but if I was offered I would certainly be going for it. We shook hands and left the office: all was going well, I was smiling. Coffee and drive home.

September 1st 2016, 5.30pm
A call from St Peter's Andrology. Could I be there at 6.30pm the next day, to check in for Stage 2 procedure on September 3rd ? This would include urethrocutaneous fistular repair with Z-plasty and fat flap, join up urethroplasty with martius fat pad, burying of the clitoris and ablation of the vagina, glans sculpting with a full thickness skin graft.

    I wasn't expecting that at all. Yes, I would be there, I said. Things were moving so fast for me. Other people were stuck on lists, but I was in again and couldn't believe my luck! This time, I was to be in the hospital of St John and St Elizabeth, London. I had never been there before, so didn't know if there was any parking. It would be a three day stay. Without notice, there was no time to do anything or make arrangements for work or animal commitments, but we would make it happen. My daughter had the animals, a sign went up at work, there was a quick text and call to family, telling them I was back in hospital and not around for a while, and that was it - packed and ready to go!

    We started our journey down to London at 5.30pm on the Friday. We had managed to find Julie a small bed & breakfast just three miles away, which was a relief because I had asked around and there is a small car park, but you can only park for two hours and after that it is £10 per hour, which we certainly could not afford. At the weekend, you can park for free on the roads nearby, if you find a space. The traffic on the way down was a pain, but as I was checking in the night before, there was no urgent rush.

We arrived at 7.45pm, at a massive hospital, a lot bigger than the previous one I had been in. We parked in their car park around the back, I gave my name at reception, and they pointed me in the direction of the ward I was going to. As we walked up the corridor we saw an open door. This was a chapel. It looked amazing and we went inside and lit a couple of candles, lovely. We came out and followed the signs for the St Francis ward, on the second floor. This was ironic: I was born in St Francis Hospital in Leicester, and now I was to be re-born on St Francis ward. That made me smile. Two members of staff at the ward reception were talking to each other, then looking down. Neither of them acknowledged me for a good while, then one turned and looked at me - not even a hello. It kind of threw me, to be honest, I had been in exceptional hospitals with very caring people and the initial impression here was not too clever. I said I was here to check in, please. "Name." I gave my name. "Room 22." I looked at her, then at Julie, then back at her. "Do I go there now?" I asked. "Yes, Room 22, over there." I was a little concerned, not a pleasant reception. We walked into the room and switched on the lights, it was cold in there. I closed the window - it was September and chilly. I turned to Julie and said, "Do I just sit here and wait?" "I guess so," she said. We didn't really know what to do, so just put on the television and waited. At 9pm no one had come to us. Then 9.30pm, then 9.45pm. We were getting concerned as Julie also had to check into her b&b. At 10pm a gentleman who looked like a waiter came to give me a menu list for my breakfast the next day. Even though I doubted I would be eating, I filled it in and asked him if anyone was coming to see me. He said he would check for me. A nurse came in and said someone would be with me shortly. It was 11pm before someone came to check me in, that was three hours of not knowing what I was supposed to be doing, with no cup of tea or anything offered. I mentioned I was cold and had shut the window. The member of staff said she couldn't put on the heating but she could bring me an electric heater, which she did. My name was taken, a band was put on my wrist, and I was told to sleep. What sort of check in was that? Julie left for the b&b; we had driven by it on our way, so she knew where she was going. She called me when she got there, so I knew she was okay. We spoke and she said she would be back with me at 7am.

I lay in bed thinking. I wasn't fully comfortable this time around, not as relaxed as I had previously been. I looked in the bathroom and the shower was inside the bath like ours is at home. I remembered struggling to get in and out of the shower, and thought that might happen here. I must have nodded off, because the next thing I knew, it was morning. I was feeling nervous and no one had come in to see me. When, eventually, a nurse came in and looked at my notes, I asked her when I would be going down for surgery. She didn't know, but said she would find out for me. She came back a few minutes later, saying I was scheduled for 12pm. I wondered how long the operation would take. I had googled it and surgery times were three to four hours. The nurse told me it would only take one hour. Oh, I thought, that's quick. I wasn't convinced the nurse actually knew, and didn't want Julie thinking I was due out, then getting worried when I wasn't. Julie arrived back and we waited to hear from the consultant, or somebody that could tell me what I was having done that day. The previous nurse came back in, told me to have a shower and gave me a little cup with some red stuff in. This was my shower gel, some kind of chemical stuff. I was feeling very on edge.

The consultant came to tell me what I was having done, and that I would be going down around 12pm. He checked all my notes, and said he would see me later on. The anaesthetist came to see me, saying she would be with me all the time and there was nothing to worry about. They were both friendly, I just wasn't so keen on the nurses this time around, who made me feel like I shouldn't be there. Next thing, a nurse walked in and called me, and I was off for my next stage. I was taken down the corridor into a small room where I met the anaesthetist. She read out what surgery I was having, but there was nothing about repairing the fistula. She went to speak to somebody and added it to the paperwork.

The cannula was put into my hand: this is it, I thought, I am going again. I remember looking at the clock: it was 11.40am. I can't even remember how I went, I can't even remember any recovery room, I just remember being back in my room, opening my eyes and seeing Julie sitting there, smiling. She leant over and kissed me, it was 5pm, so, again, quite a long time in theatre. I was still very dazed, and felt sick. I had had a sickness injection. There were three lines in my cannula, one of which was morphine attached to a buzzer. I pressed a button when I needed it, I could press it every five minutes, but it monitored the input, so I wouldn't overdose. A nurse came in and Julie recorded what she was saying. I had an oxygen tube going up both nostrils, which was a pain in the backside. The nurse explained that everything went well, I had had urethra hook up, glans sculpting, vaginectomy and a fistula repair, I had two catheters in place, one directly through my abdomen into my bladder, one in the end of the penis, and one drain. I would go home in two days with the two catheters in place, as I could not use any old bits, which were now all closed up, and I couldn't pass urine through the penis as that had a new urethra in it and needed time to heal. As I looked down, it looked like I had a nappy on my old bits, then a blue dressing on the head of the penis where they had sculpted me a glans and created me a head. They used some of the skin off my abdomen, which I called the nipple bit, to create part of the head. I had a catheter in the end of it to keep it open. On my abdomen, there had been bits either side where they had tied off when they stitched me after my hysterectomy. I had asked if these could be removed, as one was exceptionally large, and was told they would use these bits of skin to create the glans. When I looked down, I saw the large side was still there and the surgeon had taken the smaller side away. I was disappointed. The nurse said "Oh, what's this?" I said it was from previous surgery and she said "That's okay, then."

That was it, and I still have it now. My operation went well, though, so I am not grumbling. After about an hour, they brought me a cup of tea and a biscuit. I still felt sick, so I just nibbled on it. My BP was doing so much better with this operation. When I went down to surgery it was 101/65 and when I came back to my room it was 129/70. I had nicer nurses looking after me, one called Ella and one whose name sounded similar to Nosebleed. They made me smile and I felt reassured.

My notes read:
The fistula was excised and was stitched vertically. Following that, a Z-plasty was performed (This is a technique in cosmetic surgery, where one or more Z shaped incisions are made, the diagonals forming one straight line, and the two triangular sections are formed and drawn across before being stitched). The skin flap was mobilised in order to cover the fistula and the skin defect. Following that, the neourethra was marked and mobilised from the vaginal wall. This was tubularised with 4.0 Moncryl and following that, the Martius fat pad from the left side has covered the neourethra. The clitoris was skeletonized and buried. Following that, the vaginal meatus was excised and the vagina ablated with electro diathermy. The perineum was closed with 2.0 Vicryl, 3.0 Vicryl, and 3.0 Rapide. A 16F drain was left within the vagina. A 14F suprapubic catheter and urethra catheter were placed at the beginning. A full thickness skin graft was taken from the right abdomen and was de-fatted in order to be used for formation of the neoglans. A tight dressing was applied in the distal part of the phallus. The plan is for the urethra catheter to stay in for two weeks and the superpubic catheter for three weeks. The Redivac drain will remain for 48 hours and the applied dressing on the phallus will remain for one week. The aim is for the patient to go home within two days.

Julie stayed with me until about 9.30pm before returning to her b&b. I was drifting in and out of sleep. The nurse came back into me at 10pm, checked my blood pressure and administered an antibiotic through my line. They came back in at 12.30am to check my drain and empty my catheters, then at 4am to check my PCA (Patient Control Administration) in other words, my morphine pump, and how many times I had used it through the night (I had used it eight times in twenty-four hours). Each time they came in, they switched on the light, which woke me up. At 6.30am, they came to administer drugs and check my blood pressure. I felt very sore and stingy between my legs, but hadn't slept too badly, albeit a disturbed sleep. The nurse said I would be going home on the Wednesday, which shocked me as I had been told I would be going on Monday (the following day). I questioned this and she went off to find out why they were keeping me in. When she returned she apologised and said I would go home on Monday. She had read the doctor's notes, and explained she couldn't read his writing properly. This worried me - if she couldn't read that bit, what was to say I was getting the right drugs? I am sure others have great stays at that hospital, but I was not comfortable.

September 4th
The dressing over the vagina was removed, and that afternoon the lovely nurse helped me out of bed. We started off with a little walk around my room, and she said she would take me down the corridor later. I told her I was ready to go right away. I asked if was doing okay and she said I was doing really well. I was a little unsteady, but held onto her. I felt myself tensing on the way back and starting to get slightly out of breath, but I was doing it and feeling good. Once I was back in my chair, she ordered me a cup of tea and a biscuit.

Later, Julie and I went for a walk around the ward, only this time I found it hard work and uncomfortable. When I got back, I got into bed and nodded off. The pain was getting quite bad, but I didn't want to ask for painkillers as I presumed medication would be brought every four hours, as it was at the other hospital, to keep pain at bay. They had taken me off my morphine pump that morning, as I hadn't used it much during the night. I was moving in the right direction, but I hadn't had any other pain relief. When the nurse came, I asked if I had could have something and she went and got me some paracetamol, which didn't even touch the pain I was now feeling - I think I had gone too long without taking anything, and walking around a lot had made me feel unwell. Julie went to ask the nurse if I could have something stronger, and she got me some co-codamol. I didn't realise I had to ask for pain relief, I wouldn't let myself feel like that again. I was really grumpy, down in the dumps and uncomfortable. I had had a lot of surgery and no pain relief. Even if we wanted a drink, we had to go and ask. I didn't like that hospital and wanted to go home. There was no interaction, or smiley, happy people. At 9pm, the nurse arrived with more paracetamol and I asked for something stronger as I wanted a good night's sleep. She gave me more co-codamol and told me I could have a further dose at 6am. My dressings had been removed at lunchtime and nothing put back on. I wasn't sure whether this was right or wrong. I just had a pair of netted pants on, which were sticking to the glue left behind from the dressings. Top tip, buy some medical tape removing spray so, when dressings are removed, it doesn't pull your hairs so much. I am not one to moan, but surely proper pain management and aftercare is not too much to ask for? Dr R was coming to see me the next morning, so I hoped he would send me home.

5th September 2016
Discharge day. My breakfast was brought in with my paracetamol. I couldn't wait to be discharged. They had said it would be about lunchtime, after the surgeon had been to see me. Dr R came to see me at about 9.30am. He was really pleasant, but he said I had a lot done and suggested I stay another day so they could keep their eye on me. I thought he must be joking! They weren't checking on me, anyway, so what would be the point of staying here? In the end, he agreed I could go home, as long as Julie stayed with me.

He said he would get the nurses to do my discharge letter and send me home with some paracetamol. They didn't like co-codamol as it makes you constipated. The two hospitals work so differently.

A male nurse came to take out my drain. When he walked over, he caught my catheter, which pulled on me and hurt - an accident. As he was trying to get the drain out, he nicked my skin with the blade. Please, just take me home, I whispered to Julie, with tears in my eyes. I hadn't wanted to cry, but I felt myself welling up. The drain was stuck, so he tugged it. Now I did cry, this was horrendous, I felt sick, rough, really down and very emotional. He took it out and said, "That's it, you can go home now." Julie had already packed my bag. I was in there for three days and nobody had washed me. Julie would wash my face and give me a bowl so I could clean my teeth, but nothing else, so I felt dirty, too. This was the worst experience ever, and I found this stage harder than stage 1. I didn't want a wheelchair, I wanted to walk out of my room and the hospital, so we made our slow walk to the entrance to get to the car. I was so relieved to be on my way home.

Once home, we had a nice cup of tea, then I went upstairs to bed. Sitting on my 'downstairs pieces' was uncomfortable, so it was easier to lie down. Being at home was so much nicer. My pets came and lay with me, and Julie managed to get me into the shower, which made so much difference to how I felt.

7th September 2016
Julie went to open up the garage, and I videoed myself talking about how I was feeling. I was crying and hurting. The pain had got less in the last couple of days, but I was feeling lost. The catheter was still in place so I didn't need to go for a wee. I had a dressing on the head of my penis that had to stay on for a week, but there were no dressings on the old stitched vagina site and I was so sore in that area. I had opened my bowels for the first time, five days after the operation.

Julie had made me a salt bath the night before. She helped me get in, then I knelt and eventually lowered myself. It was only for about ten minutes, but was very nice. Getting out was a different matter, I couldn't even bring myself to sit upright in the bath - physically couldn't do it. My hand was still swollen from the previous operation twelve weeks ago, so I couldn't put pressure on it to push myself up. The stitches made it sore to sit, I couldn't do anything for myself. My mind was not in a good place, I was totally reliant on Julie and this wasn't me. I wanted to do things, but once again my body wouldn't let me, which left me feeling incapable, with very low self-esteem. I felt so run down and unhappy I didn't know what to do with myself. This was an operation I had waited so long for and I was grizzly because I was in pain. Bloody paracetamol did nothing. Julie called my GP and he wrote me a prescription for something stronger: co-codamol, lactulose to counter any constipation and diclofenac for swelling.

11th September 2016

One week and a day post op, I went out in the car, as a passenger. It was nice to get out of the house. I was still very sore, with a stinging, burning sensation, only getting relief when lying down with no pressure or weight on the area. The antibiotics and diclofenac were a massive help, and I had slept better. Julie filmed my bits down below, as I couldn't see them and was interested. It looked as though I had been kicked between the legs a lot of times - very swollen and bruised, no wonder I struggled to sit down. I was due back at Harley Street in a few days, so I would see what they said. I wasn't really sure what I should look like, as this time around I had not seen a district nurse, but it was bloody sore.

I had a catheter sticking out of the end of the phallus and in the abdomen, two of the lovely things to cope with. The one in the phallus bled a little, and Julie was cleaning that daily, with saline solution. If not cleaned daily, it would smell, as even after a few hours there was an aroma. Julie made a small pad to stop the phallus resting on my swollen sore bits. That collected a small amount of blood too. She was my angel, my Florence Nightingale. One of the hardest things was that taking the co-codamol got rid of the pain but bunged me up, so it hurt to go to the toilet. It was a vicious cycle.

I think I had pushed myself too hard by going to work with Julie the day before. I didn't do any work, just sat in a wheelchair we happened to have. The only time I got out was to go to the toilet to empty my catheter bag or to make a cup of tea. But I found being up and walking around made things more painful. At home, I could sit for a couple of hours then lie down to take the pressure off for a while. I knew I had to do things, but being up all day and out at night, as it was one of our children's birthdays, had been too much.

13th September 2016

Woke up feeling good! It was the day to go to Harley Street. We travelled by car, arrived in plenty of time and sat in the waiting room. It was quite nerve-racking. I was thinking that they would remove the catheter, and I didn't know how they would do that, so was a little on edge. I was looking forward to seeing my 'head' for the first time.

A consultant called us in. I got onto the couch, still feeling nervous. First, he removed the dressing from my side – the bit they had used to remake my fistula. He said it looked great and was very pleased with how I had healed. Then he took one of those Stanley blades and started cutting at the dressing on my penis. He took off the blue dressing, then continued to cut at the dressing underneath, where I had had a skin graft on the actual head. They had cut all around the penis about an inch down and rolled back the skin to make it look like a circumcised head. It looked amazing! The consultant put alginate dressing just around the skin graft, to draw any moisture out.

Then he began to take the catheter out of the end of the penis. Now that was a strange feeling. He put a non-needle syringe into the end and sucked out the saline solution that helps keep the catheter in place. Once he had drawn this out, he pulled out the catheter slowly. It didn't hurt; just a twinge and a feeling like I had just wet myself. I would not be urinating through it yet, as it had been there just to keep the urethra open. He said I was healing really well and to carry on with what I was doing. The cleanliness was great, no infections, he was very pleased with the results of the glans sculpting too. He gave me an antibiotic tablet, just because the catheter had been in a while, then said I was free to go, and should make an appointment with my district nurse to remove the final catheter after two weeks. I went home happy.

One week later I was starting to heal very well. The stitches were still in and the area was still very sore, but I was starting to walk around for longer and sit for longer without fidgeting. My mood lifted as the pain subsided, but I had found this op harder to cope with. I returned to light duties at work, and started driving the car, back to my old self again. I received a letter from the consultant saying: This gentleman's stent was removed and the dressing was also removed. The glans graft looks healthy and he is going to use some alginate dressing until it dries. He will have his suprapubic catheter removed by the district nurse after two more weeks.

After a further week I was struggling with bladder spasms; this was horrible and would have me doubled over in pain. I contacted my GP and explained what I was feeling - it was a cramping pain and felt like it was burning. Apparently this can happen when a catheter is in place. He prescribed me something called Oxybutynin, which worked wonders after the first day; I was really grateful for those little pills. I also called London and explained what I was feeling. The nurse told me to contact the district nurse to have the catheter removed, saying she would call in a week to check up on me. The district nurse I saw previously said she would remove the catheter in a couple of days. I was excited about that.

23rd September 2016
The district nurse came at 10am. We had a chat and she said how well I had done, then she pulled on her gloves and gently removed that tube that was in my belly. It was out, that was it, no more tubes! I was feeling good. I would now be urinating out of the penis, not into the bag - exciting times. I was looking forward to needing that wee. An hour passed and I knew I needed the toilet. This was going to be the first time I would be standing to pee. I went to the bathroom, I stood there, I still stood there, still stood there. Could I go? Nope, not a chance. I had stage fright, all on my own. I decided to stand there until I went. Then a dribble happened: I was overjoyed! Then a bit more, then, whoosh, it went every-bloody-where, left, right, up, sideways, it was like a showerhead. But now I couldn't stop it, either. It feels strange, because even though you are peeing out of a different place it feels like it's coming out from the original place. I always wondered why men peed on the seat. I never understood why, if you have something to aim with, it still went everywhere. Hmm, I thought, maybe I need to sit down for a while and practise in the shower until I have this mastered. The last thing I want to do is pee everywhere. I now wanted to drink everything, so it made me need to go to the toilet. It was a great feeling, standing up to pee, I loved it.

I can remember going to the shopping centre and needing a wee, so I went into the toilets and thought, yeah, first time to use a urinal. No-one was in there, I got out my piece, started to have a wee and someone walked in and stood next to me. It was as though someone had shoved a cork in the end; it instantly stopped and I froze. I felt well awkward standing there with nothing coming out. You just stand there, thinking hurry up, need to get out. As time goes on this does get better.

October 3rd 2016
I went back to full-time work four weeks post op. I was feeling great in myself and could do most things. I had a phone

conversation with Harley Street, just to check everything was okay. My aim was much better, I was getting on well, but I told the nurse that after weeing, I would dribble. She advised me to "milk it", which means making sure all the urine is out by emptying properly. I have to say, though, this didn't work for me, and I found pushing up under the testicles and underneath the penis, where the old urethra was, more useful. If I press lightly there, any remaining urine can empty. It's as if there is a little cul-de-sac inside, where urine can collect. The nurse was happy that I didn't have any problems, and said she would put me onto the list for my final stage. I was proud of how I had healed and hadn't had problems. I have been lucky throughout my whole journey.

I felt brilliant during the next few weeks. We went away for a couple of weekends, and sex cropped up. I had sexual feelings just like anyone, and we got heated one night and managed to have penetrative sex, which was awesome. I am saying this because I want others to understand how and when things work. I was flaccid at that stage, with no implants fitted, so penetration was awkward, but we found a great solution. Condoms or penis sleeves are the key. I found two condoms worked perfectly, as it gave just enough rigidity. Something we purchased from an online store worked just as well, and also gave my partner pleasure. These are things to consider during stage two, for a great sex life.

Life was great! I was back at work doing things I enjoy, and also managing to have sex, so things couldn't have been better. Time flew by, Christmas came and went, and then... Bam! A phone call from St. Peter's Andrology - could I go in tomorrow for my final stage? Wow! A late call again, but yes, I could do it. I said yes without knowing what hospital I would be at, or what surgeon it would be. When the person on the phone told me it would be at St John and St Elizabeth hospital, my heart sank, because I hadn't liked it there. However, I had liked Dr G , the surgeon, and this was my chance to be complete – I couldn't wait!

We made all arrangements as before, but this time I would only be staying in for two nights. I would be admitted on 12th January 2017, with the operation on the 13th. We drove down to the hospital on Thursday afternoon, arriving at 6pm. Check-in wasn't as bad this time. Our son took us down, as Julie had to get back because we now had an eight-week-old puppy, so she wouldn't be able to stay with me. They settled me in and the nurses came in at 8.30pm, to check my blood pressure, which was 134/84. Once I was settled in and happy, Julie and our son headed back home. I watched television and nodded off. A nurse woke me up at midnight to re-check my blood pressure. She asked if I was okay and if I wanted any medication or pain killers. I didn't understand this, as I was only there tonight because of the travel distance and had had nothing done to me yet. Why would I need medication? This made me feel uneasy and I wasn't convinced they knew what I was in for.

At 6am they told me I would be second in line for the operation, so advised me to get up and have a shower. They gave me some red Hibiscrub to have a shower with. This is an antiseptic shower gel, used before operations. The nurse came back in fifteen minutes later, saying I didn't need the Hibiscrub. She apologised. No problem, I thought, she is the nurse. Just as I was about to have my shower, the surgeon's wingman came in to see me with all the paperwork. He started to go through the procedure and it made me more and more uneasy. I know it's his job, but he was telling me all the things that could possibly go wrong. I understand why they do it, but it is frightening. He told me there is a high infection rate, with the implants, as they are foreign bodies which the body is not used to; there is a chance of losing the phallus. I thought, shit, after everything I have been through, there is a slight chance I could lose it all: that is scary!

As I signed the consent form, he asked me if I was superstitious. "No. Why?" I asked. He told me it was Friday the 13th. I hadn't realised, but I was not letting that put me off. We laughed, then he asked if I had had my Hibiscrub. When I explained that the nurse had taken it away, he said I must use it, and told the nurse to fetch more. He explained to me I should be going down to theatre at about 11am.

   I knew there were two other guys in the hospital having the same operation as me, as we had been chatting on social media, so we all gave our room numbers and I went off to find one of them. We chatted for about twenty minutes. We were both nervous, he told me he was going in last, and I knew I was second. I wished him luck and went to find the other room. I didn't expect to see anyone there, as we thought there were only three of us. But number three was also in his room, so we figured there must be a number four already in theatre. It was nice to be able to give each other support. There was just time to give Julie a quick call before I was to go down to theatre.

We had spoken for about five minutes when in walked the nurse and said: "Shay, they are ready for you." I said goodbye to Julie, told her I loved her, and walked down to theatre with the nurse. I remember we went to the anaesthetic room first, and that when the nurse touched my arm I got a static shock and I laughed, telling her not to touch down below because I didn't want a shock happening down there. I lay down on the table and was talking to the anaesthetist and another man who was putting the cannula into my hand. I asked him how long he had been doing this, and he told me it was over twenty years. I remember looking at the clock and it was 10.50am. the man put an oxygen mask onto my face and the woman started to put the drug into my cannula, just as the blood pressure cuff started to inflate. I remember that really hurting and they took off the cuff, quick. The last thing I remember was thinking my arm hurt.

When I looked at the clock in recovery, it was 2.30pm. I felt sick, so the nurse got me some anti sickness stuff and put it through my line. I was allowed to return to my room, and as I was wheeled in I saw Julie, sitting there smiling at me. It was lovely to to see her, and although I kept nodding in and out of sleep, so wasn't much company, she stayed all afternoon with me. The nurses came in hourly, to check and monitor me. At around 6pm, Julie left with the friend who had given her a lift, and I had some dinner. I couldn't eat much, I was unsettled, they checked my observations every two hours, and a different nurse came to empty my catheter bag every few hours, so each time I fell asleep I was woken up again.

The following morning, I was woken up at 6.30am, with checks and paracetamol. At 8am, my scrambled egg and orange juice breakfast was brought in. I didn't fancy anything, but I knew I had to eat, as my medication made me feel sick. I was looking forward to finding out what I had actually had done in surgery, as I hadn't been told anything. Some people have one cylinder in the phallus and some people have two, depending on the size of the phallus and what room they have internally. Some people have a pump and one testicle and some people have two, and there are different testicle implants, depending on size and how much skin they have to play with. I knew the surgeon would be in to see me, sometime, and I asked when, as I was meant to be going home, but no-one seemed to know. I had been on social media that morning, on a trans forum site, and noticed that someone I had made friends with was having his surgery in the next half hour, by my surgeon, at a different hospital. How could I speak to my surgeon about my surgery if he wasn't even in the same hospital?

At 10.30am a nurse came to take my two drains, cannula and catheter out and sort out my medication, after which I was told I could go home. I asked the nurse if he had any information about my operation. He said he would try and find out and get back to me. When he came back, he told me I had two cylinders fitted, but couldn't tell me anything else. I was not very happy as I expected to be told how things went, generally. I was guessing things went well? I couldn't even see down there. Once again, in my view, the aftercare was appalling. I never even received a discharge letter. I was given antibiotics, codeine, paracetamol, tramadol and ibuprofen to take home with me. I know codeine is a high strength pain killer, and so is tramadol, but I wasn't told which or how many or when to take the medication. The surgeon is brilliant, the hospital is just a building, so it was down to the staff, their care and training. All it needed was someone to read my notes to tell me what had been done, the aftercare needed, and the date they expected to see me again, then I would have been reassured.

When my medication was given to me, I was told I could go. At this point, I was still lying in a room on my own, just left to get out of bed by myself, having had surgery only fifteen hours earlier. I felt sick, I didn't even want to get out of bed, yet I was going home. I managed to get out of bed and get myself to the bathroom to have a wash. It took me a while, but I got there. I struggled to get dressed, though, and couldn't bend over, so did what I could, then waited for Julie to help me. But what would happen to the people who didn't have partners or people to help them? My phallus was inflated, as it was when I came out of surgery, as it needed to stay like this for one week. Harley Street rang me to say an appointment had been made for them to deflate me.

Julie arrived to collect me - not happy that I had been left without somebody to make sure I was okay. As the nurse had said I could just go, Julie packed my bag, held my hand, and we walked out of the hospital. No one came to us, and we set off on our journey back to home and normality. I am so lucky to have had these operations, so the last thing I want to do is moan about anything, but I needed to know things. I didn't even know where or if I had stitches. I received a text from Harley Street, calling me in for pump lessons, which would teach me how to inflate and deflate the penis. I had a pain in my belly, which I later guessed was because I had a new foreign body in there (a reservoir), but maybe if I had been told this could happen, I wouldn't have felt so bad about it.

Letter received 20th January 2017:
This gentleman was admitted to the Hospital of St. John and St. Elizabeth and on January 13th 2017. We proceeded with insertion of a double cylinder AMS CX 18cm+1.5cm of rear tip extender. The

pump has been placed on the right-hand side, as well as the reservoir, while a medium testicular prosthesis has been placed on the left-hand side. The patient will be discharged tomorrow with the implant semi-inflated and we will deflate this in one week's time.
I read the letter happily, as it explained what I had been trying to find out. I had two cylinders fitted and I did have a testicular implant, surely this could have been told to me before leaving hospital? Anyway, I was relieved.

During the following week it was really hard to wear certain clothes as I had a permanent semi hard-on. Unless you want to point everywhere you go, you have to pick sensible clothes, ideally baggy jeans, or joggers. I managed to get a look at down below, by asking Julie to take some pictures. My first impression wasn't really what I was expecting. I think what I was expecting was more like a sack, but what I saw, to put it crudely, looked more like the original vaginal lips had just been stitched together, with the gap up the middle. They seemed to have put a testicular implant into one lip, then put the pump inside the other lip. I messaged one of the other guys who had been in the hospital at the same time, to see what he had, and we swapped photos. His was one sac, whereas mine wasn't. I didn't understand this, as we both had the same surgeon on the same date. I now know the surgeon works with the skin we currently have. I am forty-five and the other person is in their twenties, so I am guessing our skin has different qualities. People chat about this surgery on forums, and talk about the new and old method, but when I bought this up with my consultant he said there is no old or new method, they work with what they (we) have. I originally said to my surgeon I wanted the best he could give me, which he did. People tell the surgeons what they want because they see internet pictures, but that does not necessarily mean it will work for them. The surgeons know what they are doing and know what will and won't work for individuals, so I would rather let the surgeons do their job. at the end of the day I have what I want, it works, and looks great. One thing the consultant said is that we have just been made a new penis and testicles, like a twelve year old boy starting to go through puberty. This is not the creation of a forty five year old ball sack, where it has already had thirty years to drop. Even after eighteen months, it has dropped considerably. This time round, the marks of incisions made to place the inflatable prosthesis inside the penis are either side of the groin area. An incision was also made into the old hysterectomy scar, to minimise the number of scars. This is where the reservoir tank sits inside the abdomen, all neatly tucked and hidden away. This will hopefully be the last operation I have. The inflatable has an average lifespan of twelve years, but this can be lengthened or shortened depending on its usage, and it can easily be refitted.

20th January 2017 - Appointment at Harley Street.
I arrived for my appointment, nervous, as I had heard the deflation process can be quite painful and had been advised to take some pain killers beforehand. I was called in to see a different nurse this time. I lay on the couch and she examined my incision marks, which she said were all looking good and healing well. I had dissolvable stitches, so they would be gone after a couple of weeks. She was very pleased with my results. She explained she was going to deflate the prosthetic and I would go back the next week for pump training. London is a fair way to go and quite costly to get to, but they knew what they were doing, and are highly trained, so I didn't mind the journey. The nurse explained what she was going to do:
"Grasp the tubing above the deflation block with one hand, using the other hand place the thumb and forefinger on opposite sides of the deflation block, squeeze the deflation button for about four seconds, then release it, your penis will return to a soft, flaccid and natural looking state."
Well, she was trying to get me to feel what she was explaining, but I couldn't feel anything apart from soreness and swelling. I couldn't feel the block, I couldn't feel the tube and I certainly couldn't feel any little button. I found this very uncomfortable,

resulting in me asking her to stop a couple of times. The deflate button was hard to find, even for the nurse! Apparently, the block had somehow turned around so wasn't in its normal position. In the end, I was in so much pain that she said she would try one more time then schedule another appointment for me the following week, when the swelling had gone down a bit more. She had another go, but it wasn't happening, so we rescheduled. My nether regions were on fire! When she was trying to find the button, she had one finger one side of the scrotum and the other kind of up the middle bit, which was stitched. If it had been one sack she would have been able to squeeze the whole thing. I left the appointment very sore and certainly not looking forward to returning the following week.

Over the next few days, I kept trying to feel around myself. The nurse had explained what I should be looking for, but I just couldn't feel anything. Even Julie was on the lookout. I searched the internet for advice, so I could try before I went back, but in the end I just let it alone and waited till I saw her. A lot of friends who have gone through this have said it has been sore, but has been fine with painkillers, so it was probably the fact that my button had turned around, plus the swelling, which made things painful and difficult.

24th January 2017

The postman arrived and I opened up my mail as I usually would, to find my new Birth Certificate and Gender Recognition Certificate. This was it: I was now complete and certificated. I was over the moon! This has been a very hard mental and emotional journey. You go to see your GP, then get referred to a consultant psychiatrist to see if they agree with what you're saying, then get sent for a second opinion to see if they agree with the first one. All this time your life is in their hands, and you don't know whether they will even let you start your journey. Then, during your transition, you live your new life, changing your name, which causes emotional turmoil, as having a male name, using male toilets yet still having a female chest because you can't have surgery yet, plays massively in your head. Then to change legal documents you have to go to a gender panel, where six people read all your notes before deciding whether you can have a new gender birth certificate. It is an epic journey and not one to take on lightly.

30th January 2017
I arrived back at Harley Street for deflation again, and waited nervously, as I knew how much it hurt last time. However, the swelling had gone down a lot during the week, and I had taken more painkillers, so, fingers crossed, this was going to work. It was the same nurse I saw previously, which was good as she knew how it had been the week before. I lay down and she felt around, but didn't get it first time so I thought it wasn't going to work again. Then she found it. Hallelujah! She pressed the button on the end of the block and got me to feel it. If I'm honest, I still couldn't feel it, but she could deflate me now. She squeezed the little button and there was a bit of a noise and vibration as the penis deflated. It did hurt a bit, but it was still only two weeks post-surgery. It was all done and I got dressed. She would get me a phone call organised in case I had any problems, and would bring me back in a couple of weeks for pump training, allowing things time to settle. I left feeling very relieved. I was still sore, but all was good now. I was tempted to have a go at inflating, but was a little concerned that if I managed it, then struggled to deflate, I could be in an awkward situation: I didn't bother.

I was actually feeling really good about myself, the only thing was, because my operations had been so close together and just as I was back on my feet I had another op, the weight had crept back on. Of the three stone I had lost before my first operation, I had regained two stone. I wasn't fully fit yet, but I went back to work two weeks after this operation. I struggled with lifting, so just took my time and asked for help where needed. I am certainly not one to sit still, and wanted to be back on my feet.

139

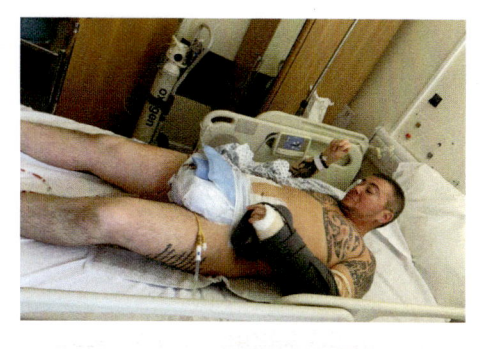

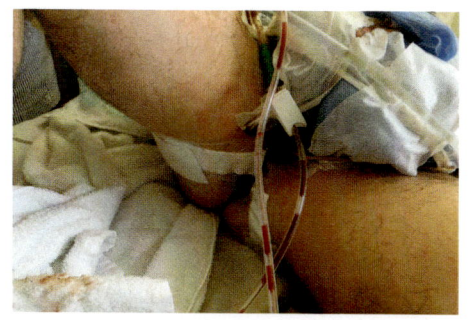

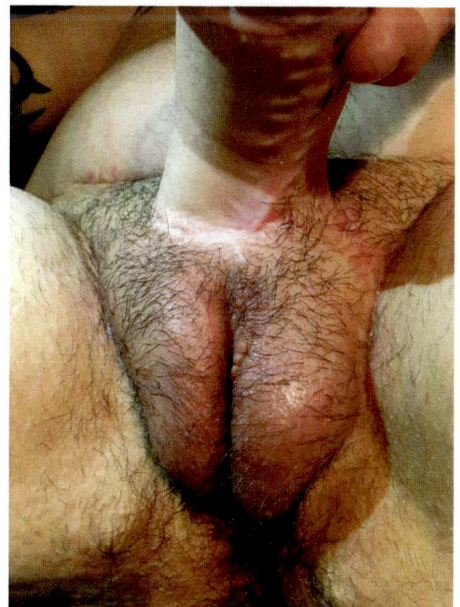

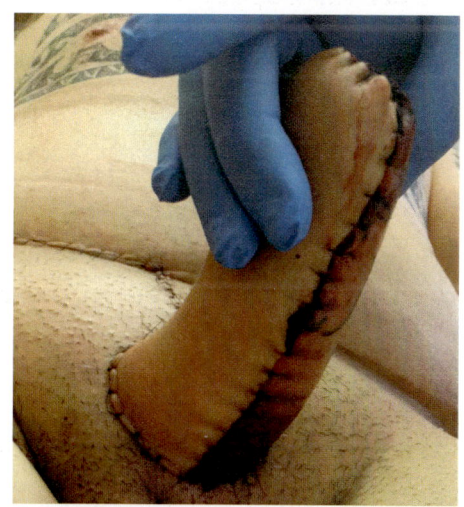

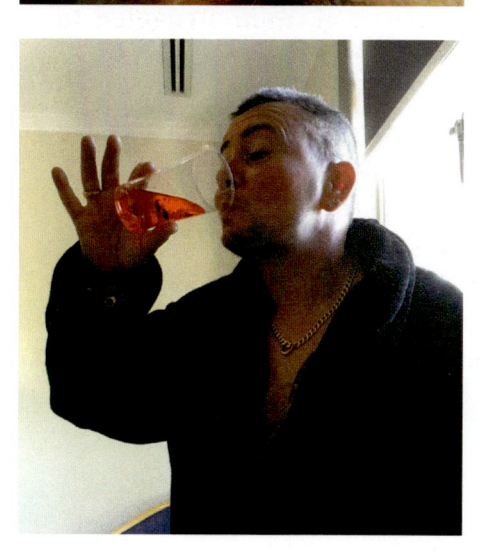

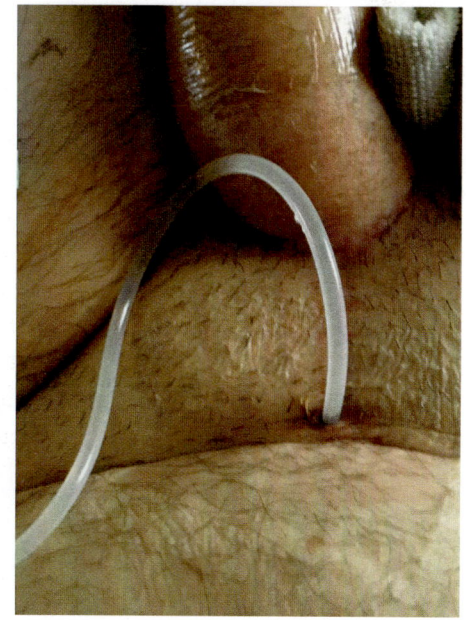

The nurse at Harley Street rang to check up on me. I was happy and healing well, so all was good. The next two weeks went really fast and I was back to London for my pump training. Back on the couch where I had spent a lot of time in the past few weeks, the nurse guided me through what she wanted me to do. With one hand I was to hold just above the block and with the other hand gently squeeze my right-side testicle, which has the pump inside. Once I had managed this and given myself a massive erection (as I am not little by any stretch of the imagination) I smiled. She then asked me to deflate, which by now I could do. Her advice was to keep practising once a day, then once I am using it fully, to go down to twice a week.

I had sex about four weeks after my op, and after talking to the nurse realised I should have waited eight weeks, to allow time for the implants to embed in the pelvic area. The sexual feeling was amazing, though, resulting in both myself and my partner orgasming, I was finally fulfilling what had been in my head all this time.

Seven weeks after my last op, I joined a gym to try and get myself fitter and to lose the weight I had been gaining over the past year. I signed myself up for some PT sessions. At first, I didn't explain to the trainer about my surgeries, as I wanted him to see me and train me as male. After a few sessions, though, I did open up to him. He was shocked and said he would never have known if I hadn't told him. The main reason I told him, was that I was starting to get uncomfortable feelings in my stomach from doing crunches and sit-ups and from being on an exercise bike for long periods, because of the reservoir in my stomach. I could feel it if I did too much, so I needed to tell him, as I didn't want him thinking I couldn't do something, or was slacking. From then on, he worked around it. I also had sessions at home with a friend who was a personal trainer.

A couple of months passed and everything was great. I had healed really well, no pains, no infections, was back at work, and had a healthy sex life. Things couldn't be any better. I had a check-up at Harley Street with one of the surgeons. He examined my hand, which was still swollen, twelve months after stage one. He seemed to think this might be how my hand would stay, and told me to try a compression glove again to reduce fluid retention. He examined my arm and was happy with how that had healed. I now had all feeling in my hand and arm, rotating was awkward, but everything was how it should be. I dropped my trousers and he had a look at my new penis. He managed to deflate me slightly, as I hadn't fully done it, apparently. I have found that sometimes, even though I deflate, it can still inflate partially on its own. He mentioned that I am on the large side and said I could go back and have this reduced, if I wanted, but Julie and I agreed we are happy with what we have. Not only that, but I have had no issues whatsoever, and do not see any reason to go back under the knife just to reduce my size. He shook my hand and said that this would be my last appointment, but they would be at the end of the phone if there were any problems. Obviously, this is nice to know.

Chapter Seventeen

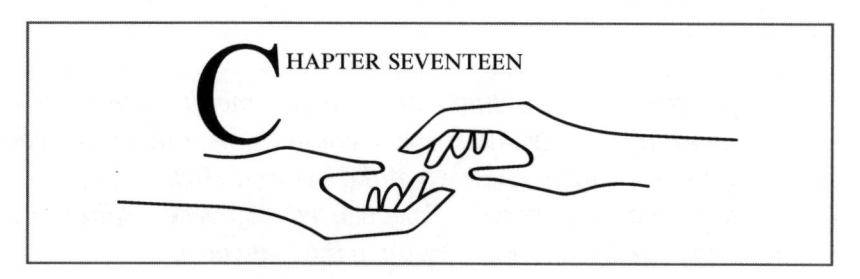

From Sally to Shay - This is Me!

I left the clinic smiling, to resume my happy life. During my transition I had spoken to an agent and I wanted to get my story out, as I had found it really hard to find information during my journey. She managed to get me a deal with 'Take a Break' magazine, and they agreed to publish my story. This was exciting; I never expected to see myself in a magazine, but if I could help even one person with their transition, it was all worthwhile. I also wanted to find people who would validate the way I felt, so I would know I wasn't alone.

My story was published on 27th April 2017 and I went to the shop to buy myself a copy of the magazine. I was shocked when I saw the front cover: "MUM'S SURPRISE – Corrie star turned me into a man!" I turned and looked at Julie; what a crock of shit that was. I was panicking now; I did not and never would say that. I had made a comment that I liked the way Shayne Ward looked and styled himself, I admired him and thought him a good-looking bloke, but I certainly did not go through transitioning because someone turned me into a man. It's a bit like a woman admiring another woman's dress or hair; it does not mean they want to be them. I opened up the magazine to see the headline: "Mum's got a beard!" I didn't like that either; this whole story was about me, but now my kids were being brought into it. I read the rest of the story and 90% was what I had said, but very elaborately written. To my astonishment, however, I was soon inundated with social media messages thanking me for sharing my story, often from parents with children wanting to transition. It felt great to be helping others.

"Just read your story... and literally broke down. I looked to my wife and said this is what's missing for me. Trouble is I'm scared what my family and friends would think. But thank you for making me realise I need to make the first step."

"Hiya, just read your story in Take a Break. So very inspirational and moving. Good luck with everything that you do x."

"Growing up I have always known I was different from a very early age. I think I was about 5 years old saying to my mom "When is my willy going to grow?" As a child I refused to wear anything girl related, never had a doll and was definitely not interested in playing with girls. When puberty hit I was devastated, my body change just felt wrong and unnatural. I was 11 years old and I think it was around this time I stopped talking because my female voice would let people know that I was a girl but looked like a boy. My parents just passed me off as a very shy tomboy which I liked because it had "boy" at the end of Tom. I had my first girlfriend when I was 15 and she told all her friends I was a lad, we split after 3 years because of people finding out the truth. She said she didn't want to be a lesbian and neither did I, I told her I was going to have a sex change but I didn't know what I had to do. I carried on with life, found alcohol and just hung around the park getting into trouble like teenagers do. I got a job in a factory with my mom for 8 years and she basically did all my talking for me telling everyone I was very shy and didn't speak. Years passed and I met my soulmate..., she told all her friends she wasn't interested in women and wasn't a lesbian but there was just something she liked about me. We had been together nearly 10 years and I asked her to help me as I was feeling depressed about not being able to talk and communicate with people, she arranged a Drs appointment. Dr said she thought I had a selective mutism and sent me to see a psychologist. I got

prescribed anti-depressants which I'm still taking today, my whole life changing for the better and gradually I became more verbal and confident. During this time, I started to spend a lot of time with my brother in law. We would go to the gym and go fishing together, he would confide in me and me in him. I told him I felt like I was in the wrong body and he said "you will always be my bro". I was so chuffed to hear this. I told him I hated this lesbian label that made me unhappy for many years. 25/4/17 I felt my whole world turn upside down, my life was about to change. I was holidaying with family in North Wales and as you do I bought a couple of magazines. I read this story by Shay Sal Robertson, OMG I felt my heart pumping faster, I was smiling from ear to ear, I was overwhelmed with happiness and started crying. I read it over and over and over again. "That's Me" I said to myself " I'm Transgender". I don't think I would have been this happy winning the lottery. Just reading the word Transgender I remember feeling a sense of relief that finally there was a word that describes me. I realised in that moment past feelings and anxieties I suffered with now finally made sense to me. I contacted Shay the next day through social media to thank him for putting his story out there. I was so excited: " What do I do now?" I asked him. He told me to make sure a million % this is what I wanted, he said I must come out to my family and friends and see my GP to get the ball rolling. I told...the next day and she was fine with it, she told me I see you as a man anyway. I was shocked and overwhelmed at my family and friends acceptance too. "Why was I so scared?" I didn't sleep for days I was so happy and excited. My GP referred me to... (gender identity clinic) but the 30 months wait for my first appointment felt like a kick in the teeth, I am 45 years old and feel like I have waited all my life for this transition to happen and felt like I had no choice than to go private, while I wait for my NHS appointment. My journey is just beginning and to be honest I can't wait to look in the mirror and say "There you are". I can't thank Shay enough for all of his help, he's made me look forward to life for the very first time. I've struggled to find much information on transitioning and have to rely on Shay, who's gone through it himself. I hope one day I can help others, like he has with me."

I also received a message from Shayne Ward's sister. I will not publish her words, but her message was lovely. Her mum had read the article, thought it was great that I was putting my story out there, and would tell Shayne. He sent me a note by post, which I will cherish.

There were so many messages, way too many to write here. I was overwhelmed with the lovely comments, which reassured me that I had done what I set out to do, by writing my story for the magazine. I thanked everybody, and even to this day people contact me to ask how I am and how things are going. I answer their questions if I can, and make an effort to stay in touch.

My agent said she thought we could get this story in the newspaper, and would see what she could do. She got back to me, saying they wanted an interview. I was excited but nervous; they made arrangements to come to my house. When they arrived, I came downstairs in black jeans and a black t shirt as I was anxious about my weight. The photographer asked if I had a shirt. I said, "I do, but because of my weight it doesn't really fit now." He told me not to worry; he wouldn't take any pictures to make me look bad, and I could keep my arms in front of my stomach. I agreed to this, and he took several pictures during the morning. I asked if he could just use some of my pictures, but he said he needed to take his own. This was on Friday 9th June 2017.

At 5am on Sunday June 11th I received a text saying the story was in that day's paper. It was also the day I was taking Julie to the airport with her aunty and friends for a week's holiday. We left the house at 7am and I drove straight to the local shop. I scanned the paper and my heart sank as I saw the hideous pictures that had gone in. I could have cried. All the way to the airport I was in shock. By the time I got home from the airport the story had gone worldwide. It was everywhere, on the internet and in every online paper. I didn't expect this at all; I just presumed it would be in one paper only. My daughter called to ask me if I knew I was on a social media site. I didn't understand how they had photographs of me inside my house. My daughter contacted them and asked them to take them down, but they had purchased them from the newspaper I had dealt with, which had taken them with my consent, so could do what they wanted with them. I began to come across some very nasty people, which resulted in me not wanting to come out of my house to buy food. My partner was in a different country and I was completely lost and upset.

The story was similar to the previous one, just more elaborate, but this time social media jumped at it, with over 55,000 comments with 8.3k shares. Truth be told, they were jumping on me wanting to become Shayne Ward. I was now getting a lot of negative comments:

"Don't worry mate we have all set a target and failed."
"Whilst you're at it, do some decorating your skirting boards are nakard."
"Shows what a sick society we live in,"
"Looks like a baldy Ray Liotta."
"Looks like Minty off Eastenders."
"I think he is mentally unstable."
"He looks nothing like Shayne Ward, hasn't he looked in the mirror, SO FUNNY! He is deluded."
"I'd ask for my money back if I were you."
"He/she looks nothing like him! My mother looks more like him than he does!"
"She looks like Andy Serkis (gollum/smeagol actor)."
"Jesus Titty Fukn christ who indulges these lunatics hide the tablets before the nut job gets home."
"Should have gone for psychiatric help before going for the knife. I like harry styles but I don't want to look like him."
"What an insult to Shayne."
"Frighteningly disgusting!"
"You weren't in the wrong body, you were not right in the head."

"Reality perverted, that's all it is."
"What a dork."

I was really struggling, I did receive some very nice comments, but more negative ones. The hardest part was looking at all the nasty things about myself and not being able to comment (as this would enable people to contact me personally) or stop it. I had spoken to my agent, who advised me to ride it out.

A letter from ITV studios was hand-delivered to my work place. The team from the Jeremy Kyle show had seen the newspaper article and wanted to interview me with a view to me appearing on the show. They also managed to get hold of my work number, and called me. I had seen the show, but wasn't interested. I told them thank you but no thank you, then I shut down shop at work and lay low at home for a few days.

I eventually came out, held my head high and carried on. After about a week my agent called me and asked me if I would be interested in appearing on the Loose Women programme. I didn't want to open myself up to more negative comments or misrepresentation, so I hesitated at first, but decided to say yes because the programme goes out live and I would be able to tell the truth. I was contacted by a guy called Jack, who went through some questions. I told him I would answer questions and discuss anything but my children; but I was on edge because I didn't know what was going to be asked. I received an email to say I would be catching a train to Euston, where a taxi would be waiting to take me to the studios. On the morning of 6th July 2017, Julie and I made our way to the train station. I hadn't been on a train since I was a child, so I was lost, but luckily Julie knew where we had to go. I was also very nervous.

We arrived at Euston and were taken to the studios. We pulled up at the gates and having looked into the car, they let us through to the back of the building. We went in through a back door and were greeted and taken to our own room, where there was a bathrobe, shower and television. We spotted a few celebrities and it didn't seem real that I was going to be with them now

- my nerves kicked in. Jack came into my room to talk about the plan for the programme, but nothing was said about the questions that would be asked. The celebrities had been prepped and it would be left to them to ask what they wanted. We were escorted to the make-up department, where I was fixed up with a microphone and they put powder on my face to get rid of the shiny glare. Back in my room, time ticked away. I was watching the programme just before Loose Women when Jack came back to say they would collect me in five minutes.

They took us both down to the studio, and when the programme went live, we stood behind the stage. During the last advert break, Julie was called on and settled on the bench with the women, and I was taken to a different position where I couldn't see or hear her. I stood behind a big screen and waited for them to give me a countdown, after which the screen would open and I would walk on. Meanwhile, they were interviewing Julie. My legs were like jelly, I had never done anything like this in my life; my heart was pounding. Here we go, they counted down, that screen opened up and everybody was clapping so loud. I looked at the audience as I walked in and smiled. They liked me! It wasn't the response I thought I was going to get. I walked over to the bench and kissed the panellists and, last but not least, my missus.

The 'Loose Women' were amazing. They spoke about how our relationship has remained so strong and how we love each other so much, and they were truly intrigued with my story; we could have carried on talking for ages. The crowd was lovely too. It was so different from the response to the newspaper article. They said they had a surprise for me, and there was Shayne Ward talking to me on a television. Wow! I hadn't expected that! I watched with tears in my eyes - it was so lovely to hear from him:

"Shay, when I first read your story I felt truly honoured that somehow I was able to help you become the person you truly are. I think you are very brave and I think you are truly inspiring. I wish you all the best for the future.."

I had an amazing day, with so many lovely people I will remember for the rest of my life. They treated me with the utmost respect, and my story was out. Even before I had left the studio, I had received over four hundred friend requests via social media, and over one hundred messages saying how beautiful we are as a couple, how lovely my story is, and thanking me for getting my story out there. People were truly interested in the truth, my truth, my story. Once again, I had messages from parents of children who were transitioning and wanted to ask me questions. This is what I wanted: to be able to show it is possible to be who you want to be. I left the studio feeling very fulfilled and happy.

A few nice comments received after the show:

"I honestly couldn't tell Shay was transgender... good looking guy... all the best for the future."

"Set me off crying, beautiful."

"Watched it today you must be proud."

"I saw this earlier, brave couple sharing their story; hopefully it will give others the strength to be who they want to be."

"Watched loose women today and seen the transgender story Shay Robertson, he really inspired me, he's such a brave person like many other trans people. I've only got as far as a waiting list for the gender clinic and all this waiting gets me down even though I know it's a slow process. I know I should be proud of the person I am and the person I will become one day but the horrible comments people get doesn't make me feel brave makes me feel like I should hide away."

"I just want to say thank you for sharing all this, it's great and go you and your Mrs bloody fantastic, epic, would so love to shake your hand one day mate."

"It takes a lot of courage to do this to help educate others, I am so appreciative, if ever I am back in London I will buy you and your Mrs a drink."

"Honestly buddy, I can't even put into words how amazing your transition is. Your results are phenomenal! I am so grateful that you have shared your story very brave thing to do, gives

me a lot of hope too, I wish you all the best and happiness in the world to you and your Mrs."
"At least we can take comfort of knowing we have an end in sight, people like Shay give me hope."
"Someone like Shay gives us guys like us wonderful hope for the future and gives me the courage to keep going."
"Thank you for sharing your story honestly. Not yet decided if lower surgery is for me yet, especially when seeing how much you have been through. Keep it up, you brave, inspirational, magical being."

The messages and lovely comments kept flowing in, and not even one bad one. The story was delivered in a brilliant way by the staff on Loose Women.

I wanted to write a book. Not really an autobiography, but more a book that people who are transitioning can follow and which helps others understand the journey.

I set up a secret Facebook page, just for transmen, with graphic pictures showing my transition. Within twenty-four hours I had five hundred followers, with people so interested in where they could see the surgical procedures, how things are created, and how things work. I was inundated with messages thanking me for creating the group and telling me how it had helped people. Unfortunately, after one month the group was taken down, and I was removed. This was so disappointing; they were medical pictures, and it wasn't hurting anybody.

Messages received:
"Thank you for your openness! I really appreciate it! Bummer they shut your group down!"
"I am looking for information regarding lower surgery, would you be willing to talk to me about it?"
"You are so open, I love it, I hope you have a good day."

"I am wondering about lower surgery, I've been on hormones for about two years, I have had top surgery and a hysterectomy, I am scheduled for a revision on my top surgery on September 12th. Would you share some pictures with me please, they are for my knowledge and interest in the process/ procedure, I will not share them or anything you share with me, with anyone else. It's purely for me getting knowledge and experience."

"Aw man, that sucks, gutted for you. You did definitely help others tho, I know I really got a lot from seeing your pics and experiences so I am sure others did to. I hope you can get your stuff back."

"your group has really helped me, I have stage one in three weeks' time and I feel much more prepared for it and aware of what to expect after seeing all you have been through. The page was amazing in my opinion, really hope you haven't lost everything forever as that would be heart breaking to lose all that."

Unfortunately, the content of my page *was* lost, but something people saw for a short time was better than nothing at all.

In October 2017, I went for a photo shoot with DW Creative in Leicester, which produced some brilliant shots of myself and Julie. I was finally in a body I wanted to be in, and enjoying my life.

153

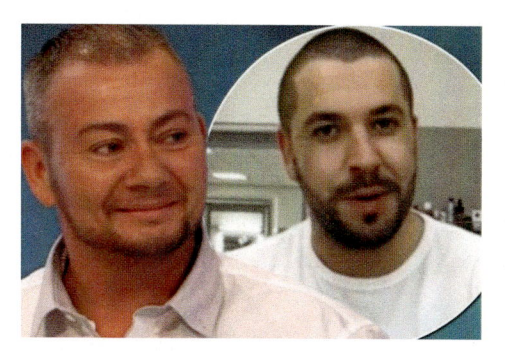

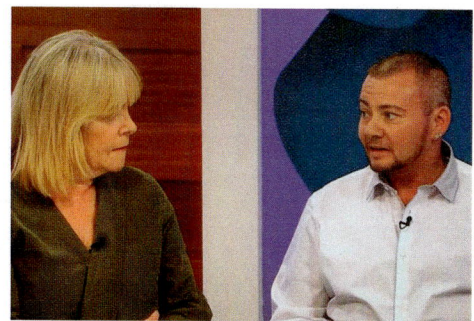

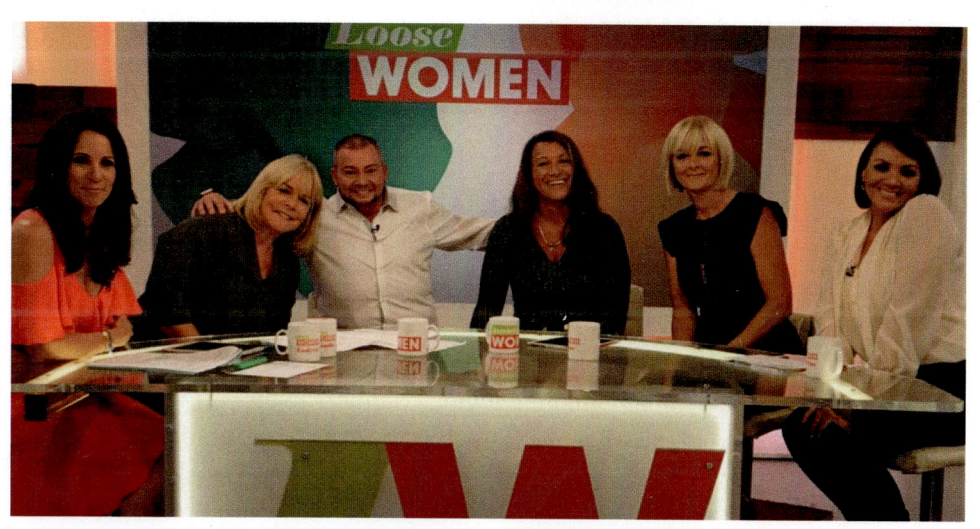

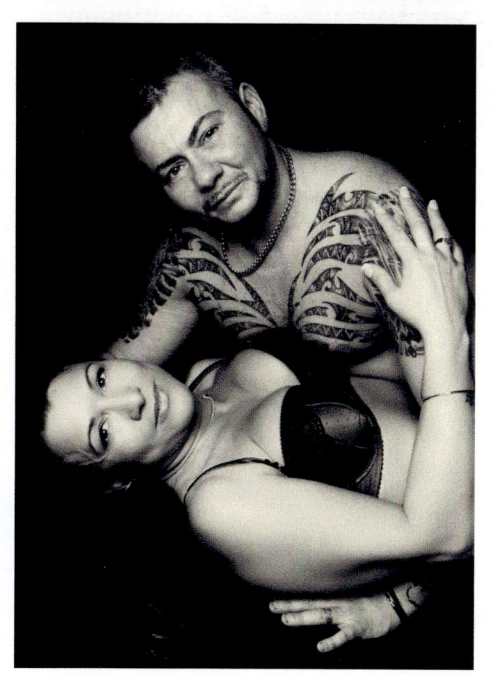

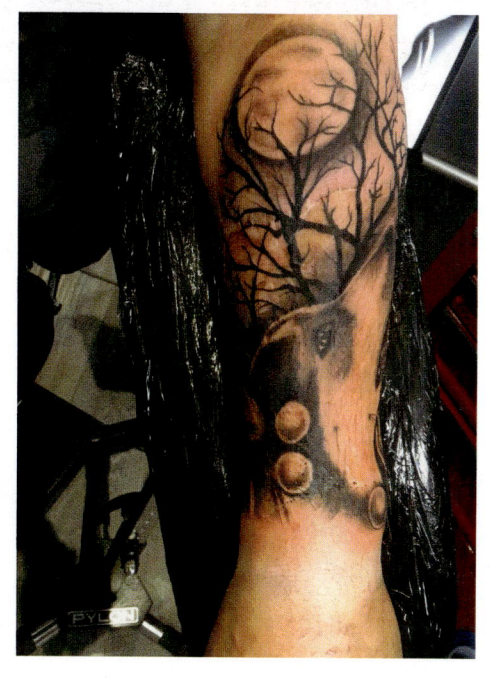

15th May 2018
Review at the gender clinic.

It was more of a friendly chat, and a chance to discuss any problems I might have had. As everything was fine, we said goodbye, shook hands and they said I would receive a letter in the post. The letter arrived a week later:

"*I met Shay in the company of his partner Julie for the last time today in gender clinic, Danetre hospital. He is now over twelve months since completing the phalloplasty procedure and has a fully functional AMS 700 penile implant which causes neither him or his partner any problems. Shay is very happy and has no regrets about treatment so far though he did meet many post-operative patients who were less fortunate when he was attending the clinic. He recognises that he has had good cosmetic result on the forearm as well as the donor site, though the "shark bite" defect is noticeable and Shay intends to have this covered with a tattoo.*

He is aware that the penile implant devices fail over time and I have shown him today one of the newer implants on the market though not I believe currently being fitted by St Peters. This is the ZSI 475 hydraulic penile implant designed specifically for transmen. It is a single chamber device and has better profile.

In terms of post-discharge care from this service, we are more than happy to see Shay again should the need arise but otherwise he is in the same position as a natal male with hormone failure. He will need to remain on Nebido 1g three monthly for the rest of his life and have testosterone levels checked along with FBC every year. Ideally, he would have a trough level of testosterone checked on the day his injection is due and then a peak level taken six weeks later. The ideal range would be between 8 and 20 nmol for trough to peak though there is considerable variation naturally and if any advice is required I am more than happy to discuss with GP colleagues in the future. His haematocrit has been steady over the last four years and it seems unlikely to me that this would rise, though it is worth watching for any increase above 0.55 as viscosity risks increase.

I completed his Qrisk 3 today based on a cholesterol ratio of 4.8 and his current weight of 85kg dressed. His BP sitting was 135 giving a relative risk of 1.8 and an absolute risk of 5.3 for a non-smoker living in Northamptonshire.

I have explained the factors that might improve his relative risk although absolute risks are still low and in particular, I think cholesterol ratio could be improved. He is returning to the gym and is considering some further weight reduction as he is carrying some abdominal weight.

Nonetheless he is a health 47-year-old Caucasian male whose risks of malignancies are now removed (cervix, womb, breast, ovary). He does not have a prostate to become concerned about. He is a lifelong non-smoker with a very modest alcohol intake and could expect decades of life ahead of him.

Management plan

Discharged to GP aftercare. Annual monitoring of testosterone levels as above. General health advice about weight and Q risk modification in keeping with males of his age. He won't need prostate examination at any time in his life as this matter may cause some confusion to future GPs looking after him. He has been advised to reduce cholesterol ratio if possible.

DISCHARGED.

I was so happy to read that letter. My journey began in 2011 and was completed in 2017 - excited is an understatement!

My life was brilliant, but I wanted a tattoo to cover my arm graft. I knew it was going to hurt, and hadn't decided on a design, but this would be the final piece of my jigsaw. I wanted a tattooist who had done scar work before. A friend recommended someone and I went along to see if he could work with my skin. He looked thoroughly and said yes, he could do that, but had a six-month waiting list. In August 2018, I went along to Lucky 13 Tattoo Studio and saw the proprietor, Jack Wilcox. He showed me a design he had created for me. I had told him I wanted it to include my three dogs, plus trees. I have to say the design was stunning.

He set to work and after two full day sittings the tattoo was completed. It was an absolutely brilliant piece of work; I would recommend Jack to anyone. I am walking proof that all transmen's scars can be covered.

My journey through transitioning has been a roller coaster, with mixed emotions and loads of surgery, but I would do it again in a heartbeat. Transitioning is not easy, and not to be entered into without careful consideration. If you read this book from cover to cover and read about my whole life, do you ask why I did this? Do you ask if it was because of a childhood upset? My answer is... NO, I did this so I could be the real me, in body and soul. I wanted to be happy in my skin, to finally love myself and be content. My only advice is this: do what you want to do, because you only have one life. Be happy, live your life, follow your dream - I did.

This is ME!

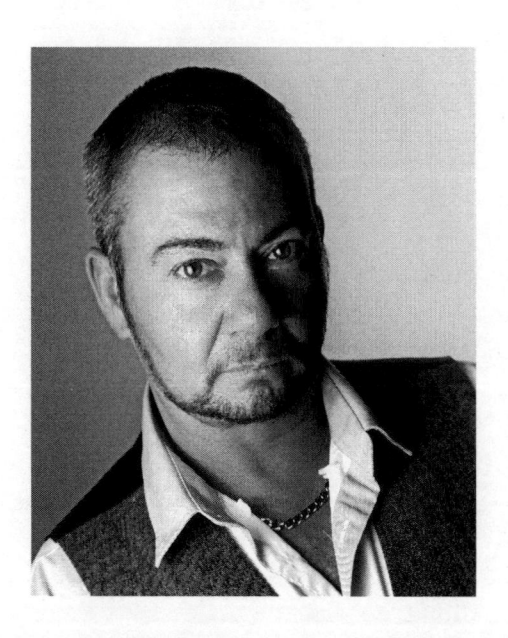

Shay

Afterword, by Julie Mclean

<u>Back then</u>
I had been in a heterosexual relationship for many years until I had a same-sex relationship in my late thirties, which I was in for a while, but only behind closed doors. It didn't feel fair on my partner at the time, or right, so I ended the original relationship, although we still remain friends. I was single for a long while after. Then I met 'Shay' through work in 2008 - a female known as 'Sal' at the time. We spoke occasionally and I felt an attraction between us, but did not act on it, as 'Sal' was in a civil partnership at the time. Unbeknown to me though, the feeling was mutual. I left the company we were both working for, none the wiser, and did not see 'Sal' again until two years later, in April 2011. Out of the blue, I received a 'friend request' via Facebook from 'Sal' saying "Hello, I found you through a mutual friend & I believe I'm working in your neck of the woods". My reply was; "You took your time!" We met up, and the feelings we had had two years prior, were still there. I had never looked at women in a sexual way, but with 'Sal' it wasn't about that, it was about the person - male or female, it did not matter to me anymore - it was the person!

Due to 'Sal' working away, we met up a week later in a Travelodge in Luton. We were talking about the looks of famous men on tv and 'Sal' was saying how she liked the look of this one and that one... By the way she was talking, I knew it was not in a sexual way but an admiring way... I looked at her and said "you want to be a man, don't you??"

Sal was taken aback by my question as no-one had ever picked up on her feelings before, even after forty years and four relationships, two of which were long-term. I was the first to see through her. 'Sal' didn't know where to look and eventually answered my question: "Yes. No one has ever asked me that before!"

Five years on, with my love and support, 'Sal', now 'Shay', has started his journey to becoming the person he has always wanted to be - on the outside as well as the inside - and no longer has to hide the real person he is inside anymore! I love 'Shay' with every part of me and will always support him in everything he chooses to do with his being. If he decided he did not want to complete the transition from female to male, due to the risks that are involved, I would understand, and love and support him just the same. But 'Shay' wants to be a whole person... the MAN that he is inside, and also now on the outside, so is adamant that he will be doing everything that needs to be done to become that person, despite the risks. And with this; I still love and support him 1000%.

I've never seen 'Shay' so happy or confident prior to starting his transition, and that is all I want for him. None of this is about me or anyone else; it is all about 'Shay Robertson' and his journey to be complete in body, mind and soul, as his real true male self! And no longer hiding within himself. I love Shay unconditionally and wouldn't change him for the world! Julie

<u>And now</u>
It's been a year since Shay had his final surgery. It has been a very emotional journey for both of us. From the very first appointment with the doctor through to consultants & hospital stays I was there taking every step with Shay, even if it meant I was sleeping outside the hospital in the car. His transition was also my transition, just without the physical changes. Would I change it?... No, I wouldn't.
It's been an amazing insight into how far someone would go and the intense trauma someone would put their body through to become someone they truly are. Watching Shay go through his

transition has been an inspiration to me; he is an amazing person and I wouldn't change him for all the world.

As well as being Shay's partner I became his nurse and carer at home throughout his surgeries and it was an honour to be part of it all.

Waiting for Shay to return from theatre was traumatic, not knowing if he would even be back with me again. Watching him go through all the pain broke my heart but it was what Shay needed to do, he was being given the ability to function and to be who he really is. It was a major step to being comfortable with his body. Despite the risks behind each surgery being extremely high, to Shay the risks were worth taking. As for me... it was a case of whatever makes Shay happy makes me happy. I would be, and wanted to be, there by his side 100000+%.

To see Shay happy and confident is all I've ever wanted and that is exactly what has happened... I've never seen Shay so content with his whole self-interior AND exterior. I have been blessed to be part of his whole journey and to have witnessed the amazing work of the surgeons that have put the happiest beaming smile on my Shay's handsome face.

I was asked by someone how I felt when my female partner told me she wanted to be a man?! My answer is: male or female I've always loved and still do love Shay for WHO he is, not WHAT he is; he is still the same person, just with a different exterior. The same eyes still look at me with the same amount of adoration, the hand I hold is still the same hand I held before, he still has the same heart full of love, the same mind & soul... He still is and always will be my heart, my love, my Shay!